the best natural homemade skin & hair care products

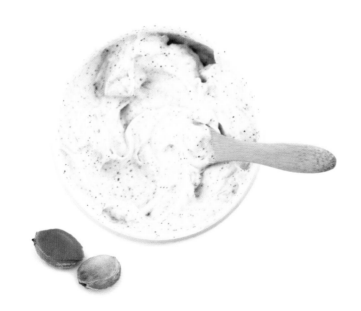

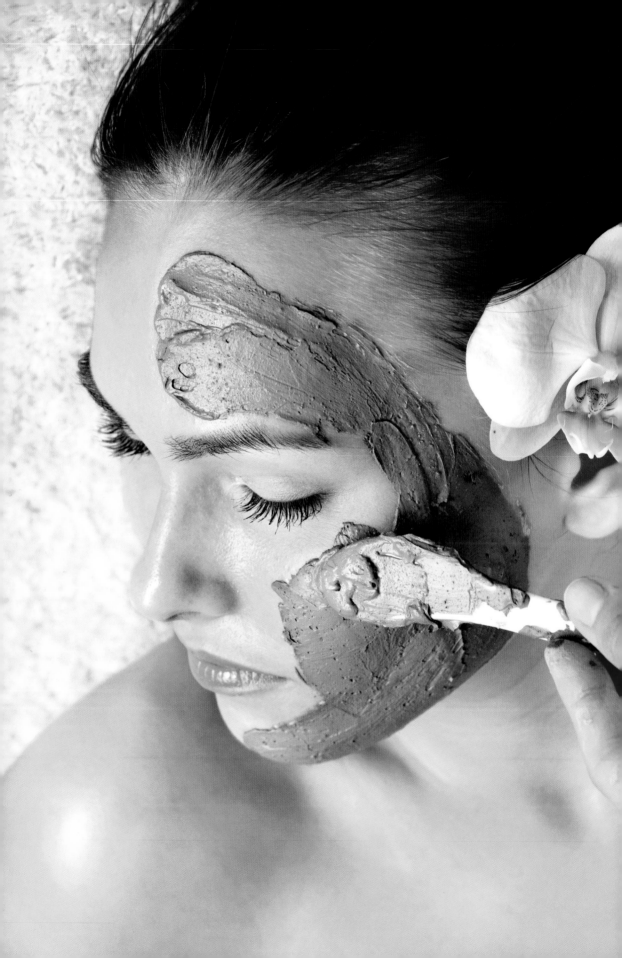

the best natural homemade skin & hair care products

175 recipes for creams, balms, shampoos & more

Mar Gómez

Robert ROSE

The Best Natural Homemade Skin & Hair Care Products
Published originally in Spanish under the title *Cosmética Natural con Aceites del Mundo*
(Natural Cosmetics Using Oils from Around the World) © 2013, Editorial Océano, S.L., Barcelona, Spain
Text copyright © 2013, 2015 Mar Gómez
Cover and text design copyright © 2015 Robert Rose Inc.

For complete cataloguing information, see page 288.

Disclaimer

The author and the publisher are not responsible for any adverse effects or consequences resulting from the use of the information in this book. It is the responsibility of the reader to consult a physician or other qualified health-care professional regarding his or her personal care.

To the best of our knowledge, the recipes or formulas in this book are safe for ordinary use and users. For those people with allergies or health issues, please read the suggested contents of each recipe or formula carefully and determine whether or not they may create a problem for you. All recipes or formulas are used at the risk of the consumer.

We cannot be responsible for any hazards, loss or damage that may occur as a result of any recipe or formula use.

For those with special needs, allergies, requirements or health problems, in the event of any doubt, please contact your medical adviser prior to the use of any recipe or formula.

Note: Natural ingredients, such as oils and waxes, can vary in color and appearance. The photos on these pages are meant to be an inspiration, not a literal interpretation. Because natural ingredients aren't processed, they may yield skin- and hair-care products that are a slightly different color or texture than what appears on these pages. That is the beautiful and exciting aspect of working with ingredients made by nature, rather than people.

Design and production: Daniella Zanchetta/PageWave Graphics Inc.
Editor: Tina Anson Mine
Copy editor: Austen Gilliland
Proofreader: Marnie Lamb
Indexer: Beth Zabloski

Cover image: Face cream with calendula flower © iStockphoto.com/evgenyb
Interior images: Blanca Vázquez, Dreamstime
Additional interior images: p.22 Baobab tree © iStockphoto.com/mtcurado; p.25 Baobab fruit © iStockphoto.com/ KarelGallas; p.35 Ylang-ylang flower © iStockphoto.com/thawats; p.38 Vitamin E capsule © iStockphoto.com/4kodiak; p.39 Fine sea salt © iStockphoto.com/Maya Kovacheva Photography; p.47 Geraniums © iStockphoto.com/BertBeekmans; p.48 Orange cream © iStockphoto.com/bluehill75; p.54 Macadamia nuts © iStockphoto.com/pengpeng; p.61 Sesame oil © iStockphoto.com/Alleko; p.66 Ginger and rosemary © iStockphoto.com/dionisvero; p.80 Chamomile flowers © iStockphoto.com/Jasmin Awad; p.83 Rosemary sprig © iStockphoto.com/Maartje van Caspel; p.86 Safflowers © iStockphoto.com/hichako; p.96 Safflower (single) © iStockphoto.com/pressdigital; p.100 Evening primroses © iStockphoto.com/epantha; p.103 Evening primrose oil capsules © iStockphoto.com/aodaodaod; p.105 Lavender sprigs © iStockphoto.com/KariHoglund; p.111 Evening primrose with bottle © iStockphoto.com/PicturePartners; p.112 Babassu oil © iStockphoto.com/Chris Gramly; p.119 Babassu cream © iStockphoto.com/brebca; p.123 Green clay powder © iStockphoto.com/og-vision; p.124 Chamomile flower © iStockphoto.com/ValentynVolkov; p.140 Black cumin seeds © iStockphoto.com/lvenks; p.143 Rosemary and thyme © iStockphoto.com/jirkaejc; p.150 Andiroba oil © iStockphoto.com/ Surakit Hartongkul; p.161 Rose hips © iStockphoto.com/Piksel; p.163 Rose water © iStockphoto.com/longtaildog; p.166 Red grapes © iStockphoto.com/mauhorng; p.169 Bergamots © iStockphoto.com/slallison; p.170 Pumpkin with seeds © iStockphoto.com/susabell; p.173 Pumpkin stack © iStockphoto.com/Moncherie; p.180 Hemp seeds © iStockphoto.com/Alasdair Thomson; p.183 Face cream and lavender buds © iStockphoto.com/de-kay; p.185 Lavender flowers © iStockphoto.com/matka_Wariatka; p.189 Hemp seeds and leaves © iStockphoto.com/Vitalina Rybakova; p.193 Mallow flower © iStockphoto.com/Volga2012; p.198 Jojoba sprig and seeds © iStockphoto.com/mashuk; p.207 Shea butter and nuts © iStockphoto.com/Elenathewise; p.208 Shea nuts and sprig © iStockphoto.com/luisapuccini; p.209 Rosemary oil and sprig © iStockphoto.com/ marilyna; p.210 Bitter almonds © iStockphoto.com/pilipphoto; p.220 Apricot © iStockphoto.com/connect11; p.224 Peanuts © iStockphoto.com/ FotografiaBasica; p.227 Hand cream © iStockphoto.com/S847; p.229 Peanuts in shell © iStockphoto.com/Rodrusoleg; p.232 Sesame oil and seeds © iStockphoto.com/tashka2000; p.242 Prickly pears © iStockphoto.com/Ockra; p.248 Tamanu oil with flower © iStockphoto.com/ Gubcio; p.256 Pequi oil with dropper © iStockphoto.com/yangna; p.259 Cream with avocado © iStockphoto.com/AGorohov; p.260 Sunflower © iStockphoto.com/Olaf Simon; p.264 Oats © iStockphoto.com/AvalonStudio_WojciechKryczka; p.266 Soybean oil and soybeans © iStockphoto.com/ ShashikantDurshettiwar; p.269 Lemon with dropper © iStockphoto.com/matka_Wariatka; p.270 Hazelnuts © iStockphoto.com/dionisvero

The publisher gratefully acknowledges the financial support of our publishing program by the Government of Canada through the Canada Book Fund.

Published by Robert Rose Inc.
120 Eglinton Avenue East, Suite 800
Toronto, Ontario, Canada M4P 1E2
Tel: (416) 322-6552 Fax: (416) 322-6936
www.robertrose.ca

Printed and bound in Canada

1 2 3 4 5 6 7 8 9 TCP 23 22 21 20 19 18 17 16 15

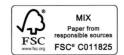

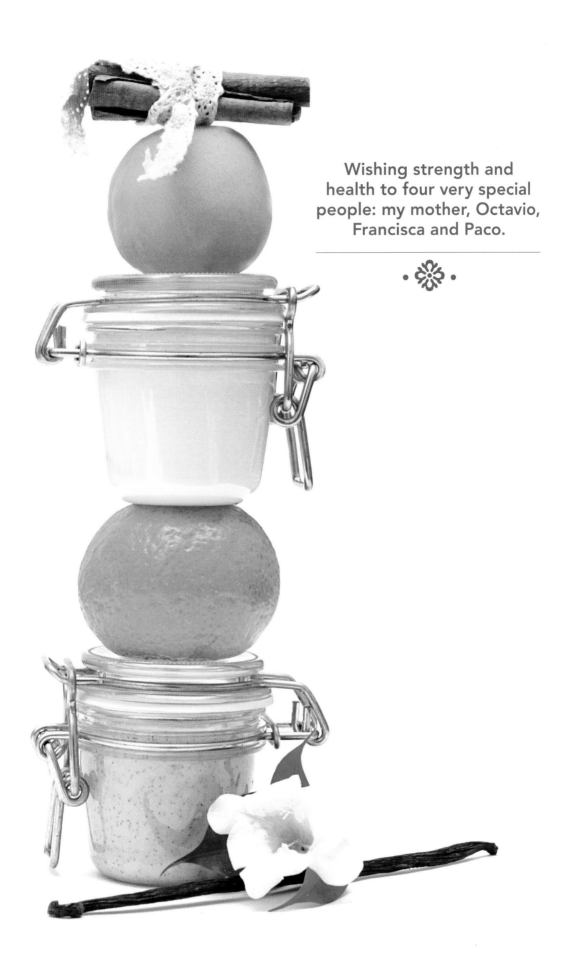

Wishing strength and
health to four very special
people: my mother, Octavio,
Francisca and Paco.

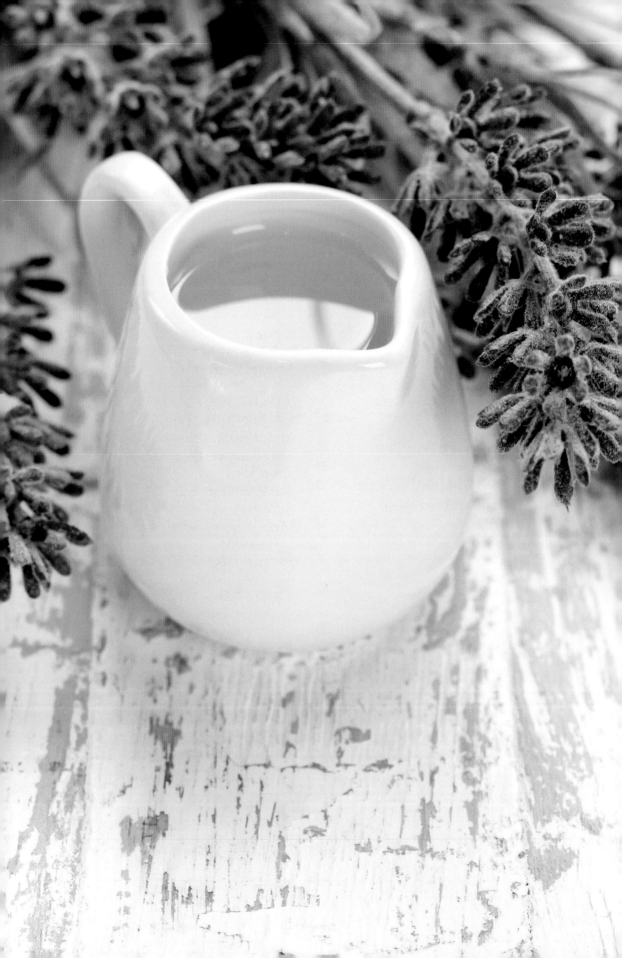

Contents

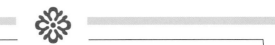

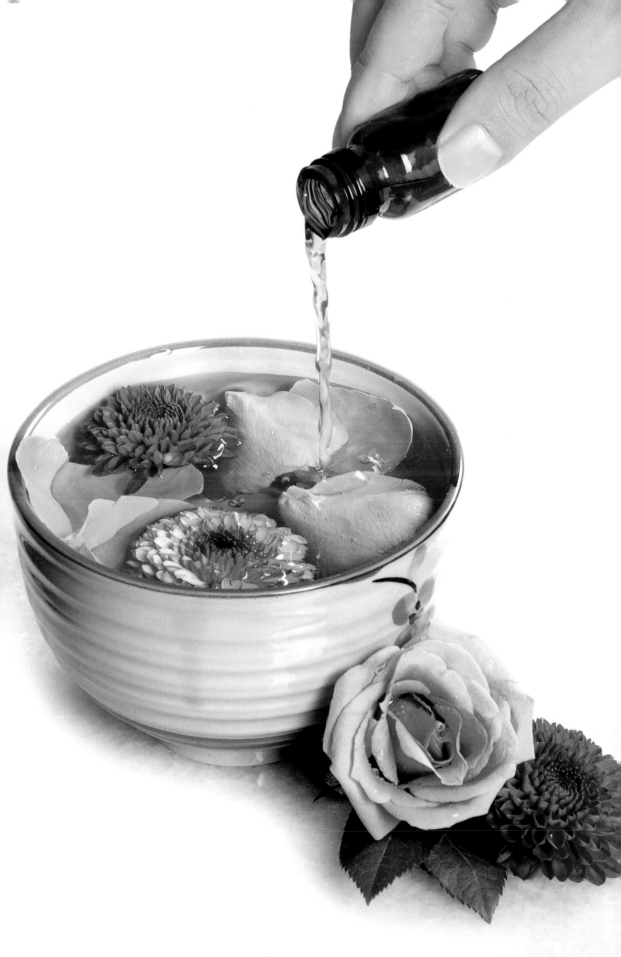

Introduction

This book is all about oils from around the world. Each has a unique set of therapeutic properties, and each functions in a different way than other oils. One may be excellent for treating dry skin, while another may help tame oily skin, and so on. In each of my skin- and hair-care recipes, I have used the oil that has the best characteristics to ensure the desired outcome. I have included many formulas to treat all types of skin. Many of the oils may not be familiar at first, but I am sure that it will not be long before they receive the recognition they deserve, just as aloe vera, tea tree oil and other natural skin-care ingredients have in recent years.

The formulas I've created, especially those used to make creams, call for a number of the same ingredients. A cream contains two main parts: the oil portion and the water portion. The oil, or fatty, portion varies from recipe to recipe. If you use a different oil (or oil mixture) than the one called for in the ingredient list, the formula will change completely, both in texture and in therapeutic properties, even if all of the other ingredients in the recipe are the same. The water part of the formula is also variable — you can use mineral water, floral waters of all kinds or even herbal infusions. Most of my creams contain Lanette wax (see box, page 15), which serves as an emulsifier, enabling the oil and water portions of the recipe to mix and form a smooth texture. This wax is one of the most gentle and effective emulsifiers you can find. The recipes also call for natural preservatives in the form of powdered citric acid and ascorbic acid (also known as vitamin C).

Good-quality essential oils can be quite pricey. Therefore, I have tried to use no more than 20 different kinds for the recipes in this book. Of course, there are many wonderful essential oils on the market, but by simplifying the formulas and using many of the same essential oils, I've ensured that you do not have to spend a lot on these ingredients alone. The advantage of essential oils is that they are extremely versatile and can be used in many recipes for skin- and hair-care products, not just the ones you find here.

Finally, a small but important piece of advice. Every two to three months, be sure to change the creams or oils you use. Your skin will get used to one formula; no matter how good it may be, it will end up losing its effectiveness. Switch to a different formula that is suitable for your needs or skin type to continue experiencing the benefits. This applies to shampoos, too.

Tip

It is important to be safety-conscious and clean when preparing and storing your homemade skin- and hair-care products. Before you start, make sure to disinfect all of the utensils, bottles and jars you use. A little splash of rubbing alcohol wiped all over the equipment then dried off with a paper towel is plenty to ensure a sanitary start. Frequent, thorough hand washing is always a good idea when preparing homemade creams, oils and other skin- and hair-care products.

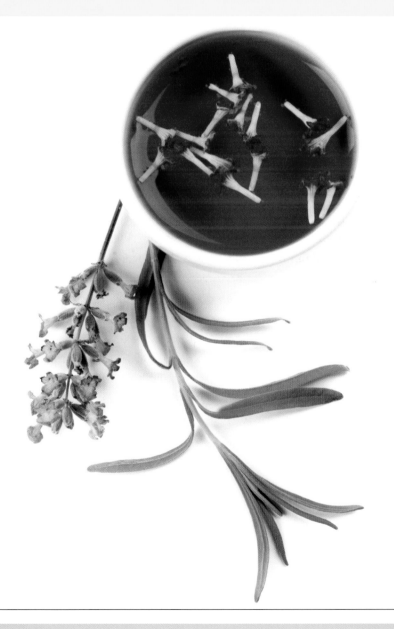

The Basic Formulas

All of the recipes in this book come with simple-to-follow instructions. But before you dig in to the process of making a face cream or a shower gel, it's a great idea to get an overview of the process. Here are general instructions for making the main types of skin- and hair-care formulas you'll find in this book (other types, such as masks, exfoliants and restorers, vary, so check out the specific recipe you're interested in). I've included how-tos, storage information and handy tips to help you get started.

Making Creams and Ointments

1. First, weigh all of the recipe ingredients (see How to Weigh Ingredients, page 17). You will need two saucepans: one to heat oils and solid fats, and the other to heat water-based liquids. Place the base oil(s) or fat(s) called for in the recipe — such as shea butter, cocoa butter, Lanette wax, beeswax or lanolin — in a saucepan and heat over low heat. When all the ingredients have melted but before they have overheated or begun to smoke, remove the pan from the heat; keep warm.

2. Pour the water-based ingredients — such as mineral water, orange flower water, rose water, infusion or witch hazel — into a separate saucepan and heat until lukewarm. Using a wooden spoon, stir in the citric acid and ascorbic acid powders until dissolved.

3. Stir the water-based mixture into the oil mixture. The two preparations — the oils and melted fats, and the water-based liquids — should be at about the same temperature so the mixture can emulsify properly. Using a hand mixer, beat the mixture at low speed for 1 to 2 minutes. Let stand for 10 minutes.

4. After letting the cream stand, but while the mixture is still fluid, stir in any liquid glycerin, essential oils, collagen or vitamins called for in the recipe. Using a hand mixer, beat at high speed for 1 minute. The cream or ointment is now ready.

5. Pour or spoon the mixture into glass jars and let cool. It is normal for the mixture to be quite liquid at this point. The cream will reach its final, correct consistency in the jar, after it is allowed to cool completely. Ointments will be somewhat thicker when finished.

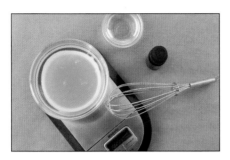
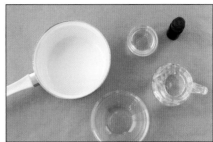

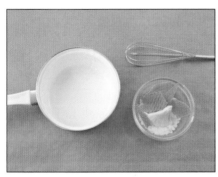
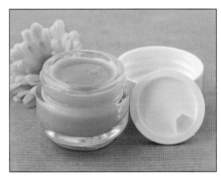

Storing Creams and Ointments

Homemade beauty creams and ointments will last for several months. If you have made more than you will use in that time, I recommend storing the excess in the refrigerator. You can make a large jarful and keep it in the refrigerator, transferring a portion to a smaller jar as often as needed. Creams and ointments should not be stored in plastic jars.

What Is Lanette Wax?

This emulsifying wax is a trademarked blend of ingredients used to bind water with oil in an emulsion. It is commonly used as a component of creams and ointments to make them smooth and uniform. It also helps them stay together so they don't separate as they stand. There are many brands and varieties of emulsifying wax on the market, but this is my favorite for homemade creams.

Making Oils

1. First, weigh all of the recipe ingredients (see How to Weigh Ingredients, opposite).

2. Pour them into a small glass bottle and seal tightly.

3. Shake gently to combine. It could not be any easier!

Tips for Making Oils

For the base oils (soybean, sesame, safflower, etc.), extra-virgin or virgin oils made from the first cold pressing are best. Essential oils must be 100% pure. Do not confuse them with artificial (synthetic) scents or oils, or essences used in fragrance burners or lamp rings.

Always use glass bottles to store homemade oils. Plastic bottles can absorb the essential oils contained in these recipes. They may also change color, or, worse still, release harmful substances into your mixture.

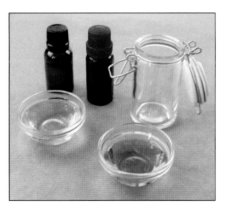
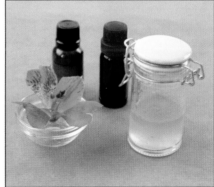

Storing Oils

Homemade oils will last for several months. Keep all oils, especially essential oils, out of direct sunlight; they are sensitive to light and may lose many of their beneficial properties if not kept in a dark place. Bottles should never be left uncapped, because the volatile oils will evaporate.

How to Weigh Ingredients

- When making body-care products, proper measurements are important. For these recipes, most of the ingredients are measured by weight, not volume, for accuracy.

- Scales come in a variety of styles. Buy a digital scale that weighs in 0.1-oz or 1 g increments. If you're using imperial measurements instead of metric, a scale that reads in increments of 0.01 oz is a much better choice for these recipes, which sometimes require very tiny amounts of ingredients, especially in the case of essential oils.

- Precision is important, so choose a scale that is accurate to within 0.1 oz or 1 g — or even better, to within 0.01 oz or 0.5 g. With it, you will be able to precisely weigh the required ingredients to make the most luxurious formulas.

- Look for a scale that has a tare button, as well. This allows you to place a bowl or other receptacle on the scale, then "zero" the scale so that it weighs only the contents. It makes the process much easier.

Making Shampoos

1. First, weigh all of the recipe ingredients (see How to Weigh Ingredients, above). Then, prepare the infusion. Place the plant ingredient called for — such as sage or rolled oats — in a bowl. In a saucepan, bring the amount of mineral water called for in the recipe to a boil, then pour it over the plant ingredient. Cover and let steep for 10 minutes.

2. Using a fine-mesh sieve lined with cheesecloth, strain the infusion into a clean bowl. Let cool completely.

3. Pour the cooled infusion, the coco betaine and the remaining ingredients into a bottle. Shake gently to combine, and the shampoo is ready to use.

4. If your hair is very dry, you can add about 1 oz (30 g) liquid glycerin, a moisturizing ingredient, to your shampoo if you wish.

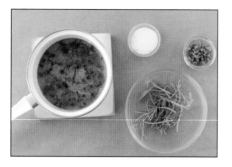

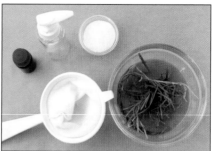

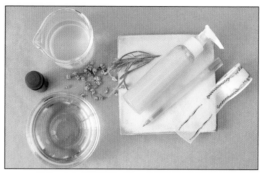

Make More or Less

You can easily adjust these recipes to make different amounts. Simply multiply or divide the amounts of the ingredients proportionately. For example, to double the yield of a recipe, just double the ingredients.

Storing Shampoos

Homemade shampoos will keep for up to three months. Gently shake the shampoo just before using, because the oils will rise to the top as the mixture stands.

Cautions

The recipes in this book are not a substitute for medical prescriptions. All recipes use natural ingredients, but bear in mind that some people may be allergic to certain substances. Before using any of the recipes, first check for sensitivity on a small patch of skin. Formulas that contain essential oils should not be used on children under six months of age.

Making Gels

1. First, weigh all of the recipe ingredients (see How to Weigh Ingredients, page 17). Pour the amount of water called for in the recipe into a saucepan. Add the amount of chopped glycerin soap base called for (the soap is sold in bars ranging in size from 1 lb to 3½ lbs/500 g to 1.75 kg). Heat the mixture over low heat until the soap base is dissolved.

2. Let soap mixture cool. Stir in the remaining ingredients.

3. Transfer the finished gel to a pump dispenser for convenience.

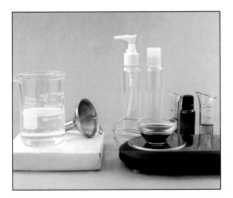
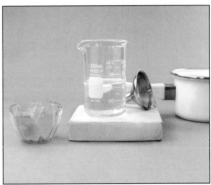

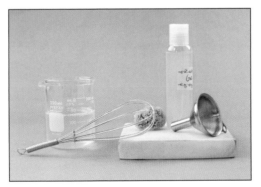

Storing Gels

Homemade gels will keep for up to three months. Gently shake the gel just before using, because the oils will rise to the top as the mixture stands.

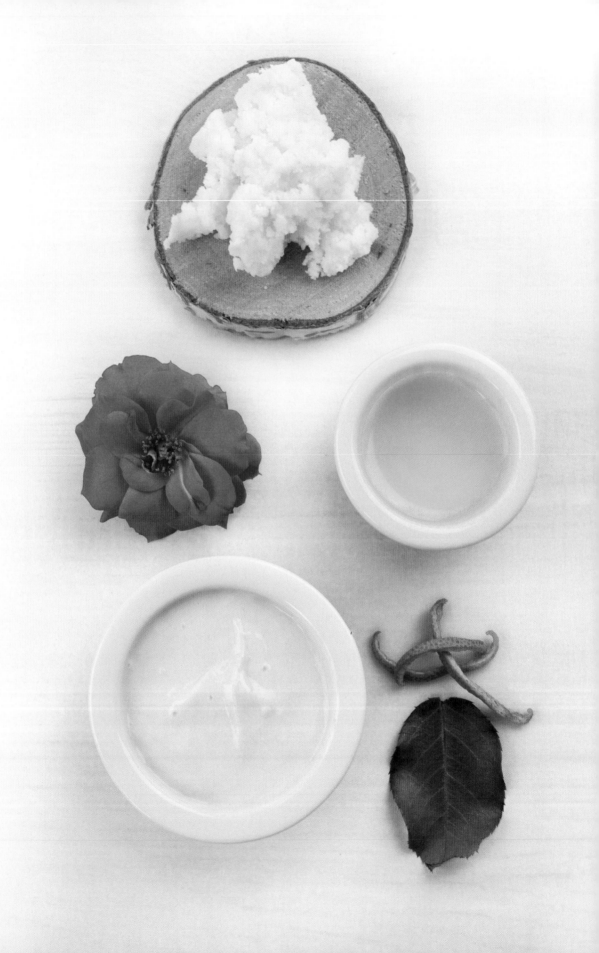

The Recipes

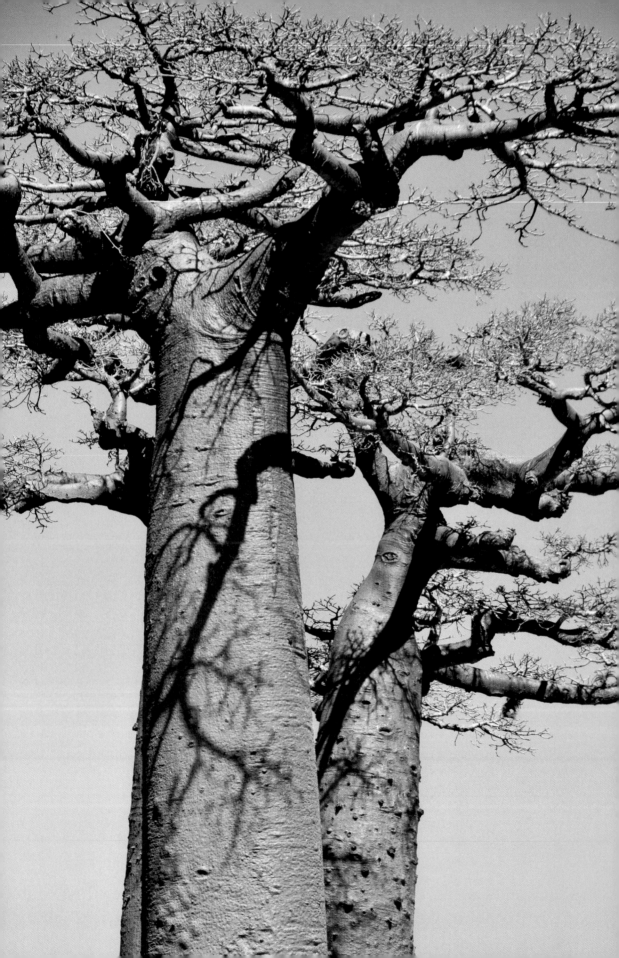

Baobab Oil

Baobab oil mixes easily with other oils, so it is terrific in cream formulas; it makes them easy to absorb and adds a pleasant, silky texture.

This wonderful oil comes from Africa. The baobab is one of the oldest trees found on the African savannas. Many are reported to have reached the age of 1,000 years or more — and some anecdotal evidence suggests that a few may be more than 2,000 years old.

According to legend, the baobab was the most splendid and beautiful of all the trees. Humans, animals and even other trees admired it; the gods, too, noticed the beauty of its strong branches, the color and fragrance of its flowers and, above all, the hard wood of its trunk. Because it was so beautiful and useful, the gods gave it the gift of long life. The baobab proudly began to grow and grow.

It grew so tall that its branches shaded the other trees and kept them from growing. Animals that walked under it were frozen in place. Eventually, the tree blocked out the sun, so any plant underneath it died. Swollen with pride, the baobab continued to grow, calling out to the gods that soon it would be as tall as they were.

The tree's audacity angered the gods, and they cursed it so that it would grow upside down. Its beautiful flowers and long branches were buried forever. The part above ground grew in the shape of roots.

For many centuries, African people have used all of the products that this great tree offers them. Its parts are used for food, and to make medicine and beauty products. Even the shells that surround its fruit are used as fuel for everyday household and cooking fires.

Baobab seeds are rich in vitamins A, B, C, D and E, and essential fatty acids. The oil extracted from the seeds nourishes the skin and is used to combat premature wrinkles and free radical damage. It is said to promote tanning and is soothing when applied after shaving or other types of hair removal, when the skin tends to be red and tender. Baobab oil restores balance to the skin, and can also be applied to the ends of the hair to prevent dryness and split ends. It is also highly recommended for use during body and face massages.

Baobab Anti-Wrinkle Face Cream

This cream helps prevent wrinkles, and can also reduce the appearance of wrinkles that are already present.

Best for: Mature, damaged or very dry skin

Tip: Look for chunks or blocks of pure cocoa butter at cosmetic-supply stores. If you're using a large amount in a recipe, chop it up before adding it to the saucepan so it will melt more quickly.

Note: Exact measurements are important when you're making skin- and hair-care products. Turn to page 17 for how-tos.

1 oz	baobab oil	30 g
0.35 oz	jojoba oil	10 g
0.35 oz	cocoa butter (see tip, at left)	10 g
0.2 oz	Lanette wax (see box, page 15)	6 g
4.9 oz	mineral water	140 g
2	pinches citric acid powder (see box, page 27)	2
2	pinches ascorbic acid powder	2
30	drops geranium essential oil	30

1. Combine baobab oil, jojoba oil, cocoa butter and Lanette wax in a saucepan. Heat over low heat just until ingredients are completely melted. Remove from heat and keep warm.

2. Pour mineral water into a separate saucepan. Heat until lukewarm. Using a wooden spoon, stir in citric acid and ascorbic acid until dissolved.

3. Stir mineral water mixture into oil mixture. Using a hand mixer, beat at low speed for 1 to 2 minutes. Let stand for 10 minutes.

4. Stir in geranium essential oil. Using a hand mixer, beat at high speed for 1 minute.

5. Pour or spoon mixture into glass jars. Let cool.

Baobab: A New Superfood

The fruit of the baobab tree has recently become a popular nutritional supplement. The pulp is dried and ground into a fine golden powder that can be added to beverages, such as smoothies, or recipes. It has a sweet-tart taste and contributes many vitamins and minerals.

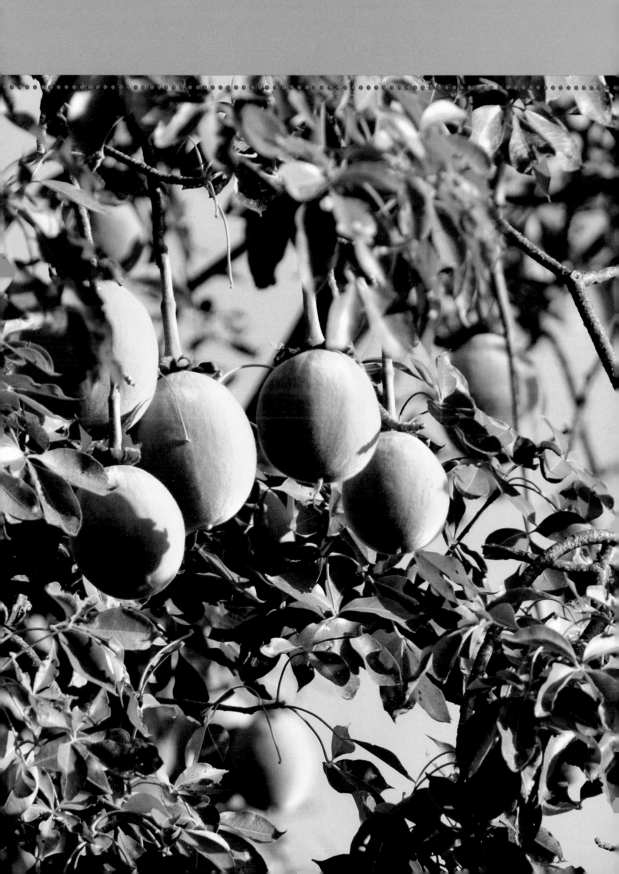

Baobab Moisturizing Face Cream

This easily absorbed cream is ideal for people of all ages. It helps protect the skin in the winter and prevents it from drying out in the summer, too.

Best for: Normal or combination skin

Tips: Rose water is often used in Middle Eastern and Mediterranean cooking. Look for it in Middle Eastern grocery stores and some well-stocked supermarkets.

The essential oils you use for skin- and hair-care products must be 100% pure. Don't use synthetic scents or oils, or essences used in fragrance burners or lamp rings.

Note: Exact measurements are important when you're making skin- and hair-care products. Turn to page 17 for how-tos.

0.35 oz	baobab oil	10 g
0.2 oz	Lanette wax (see box, page 15)	6 g
0.15 oz	cocoa butter	4 g
6.3 oz	rose water (see tips, at left)	180 g
2	pinches citric acid powder (see box, page 27)	2
2	pinches ascorbic acid powder	2
6	drops myrrh essential oil (see tips, at left)	6

1. Combine baobab oil, Lanette wax and cocoa butter in a saucepan. Heat over low heat just until ingredients are completely melted. Remove from heat and keep warm.

2. Pour rose water into a separate saucepan. Heat until lukewarm. Using a wooden spoon, stir in citric acid and ascorbic acid until dissolved.

3. Stir rose water mixture into oil mixture. Using a hand mixer, beat at low speed for 1 to 2 minutes. Let stand for 10 minutes.

4. Stir in myrrh essential oil. Using a hand mixer, beat at high speed for 1 minute.

5. Pour or spoon mixture into glass jars. Let cool.

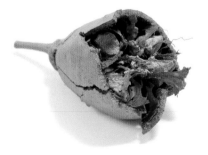

Baobab Nourishing Face Cream

This cream is highly recommended as a base under makeup. It creates a smooth, healthy surface that feels comfortable.

Best for: All skin types

Tip: Store essential oils in a cool, dark place to preserve their healing compounds. Light exposure weakens them.

Note: Exact measurements are important when you're making skin- and hair-care products. Turn to page 17 for how-tos.

0.5 oz	baobab oil	15 g
0.2 oz	Lanette wax (see box, page 15)	6 g
0.1 oz	cocoa butter	3 g
6 oz	witch hazel	170 g
2	pinches citric acid powder (see box, below)	2
2	pinches ascorbic acid powder	2
0.18 oz	rose hip seed oil	5 g
10	drops geranium essential oil (see tip, at left)	10

1. Combine baobab oil, Lanette wax and cocoa butter in a saucepan. Heat over low heat just until ingredients are completely melted. Remove from heat and keep warm.

2. Pour witch hazel into a separate saucepan. Heat until lukewarm. Using a wooden spoon, stir in citric acid and ascorbic acid until dissolved.

3. Stir witch hazel mixture into oil mixture. Using a hand mixer, beat at low speed for 1 to 2 minutes. Let stand for 10 minutes.

4. Stir in rose hip seed oil and geranium essential oil. Using a hand mixer, beat at high speed for 1 minute.

5. Pour or spoon mixture into glass jars. Let cool.

What Are Citric Acid and Ascorbic Acid?

These two ingredients are added to cream and ointment recipes to preserve them and keep bacteria or mold from growing. Citric acid is a very tart powder made by fermenting fruit sugars. The acid is present in citrus fruits and gives them their sour taste. Ascorbic acid is better known as vitamin C. This antioxidant vitamin is found in citrus fruits and many green vegetables. Both acids are used as food additives, as well as ingredients in skin- and hair-care formulas. You can buy them at cosmetic-supply stores, and some supermarkets or bulk-food stores.

Baobab and Orange Moisturizing Body Cream

The essential feature of this body cream is that it absorbs readily without making your skin feel oily. It also smells heavenly.

Best for: All skin types

Tips: Orange flower water is also called orange blossom water. It's easy to find in Middle Eastern grocery stores and some well-stocked supermarkets, where it's sold for use in cooking.

Liquid glycerin is a moisturizing ingredient often included in cosmetics, soaps, shampoos and creams. You'll find small bottles of it at drugstores, but cosmetic-supply stores sell larger bulk amounts.

Note: Exact measurements are important when you're making skin- and hair-care products. Turn to page 17 for how-tos.

0.7 oz	baobab oil	20 g
0.4 oz	Lanette wax (see box, page 15)	12 g
0.35 oz	cocoa butter	10 g
11.6 oz	orange flower water (see tips, at left)	330 g
4	pinches citric acid powder (see box, page 27)	4
4	pinches ascorbic acid powder	4
1 oz	liquid glycerin (see tips, at left)	30 g

1. Combine baobab oil, Lanette wax and cocoa butter in a saucepan. Heat over low heat just until ingredients are completely melted. Remove from heat and keep warm.

2. Pour orange flower water into a separate saucepan. Heat until lukewarm. Using a wooden spoon, stir in citric acid and ascorbic acid until dissolved.

3. Stir orange flower water mixture into oil mixture. Using a hand mixer, beat at low speed for 1 to 2 minutes. Let stand for 10 minutes.

4. Stir in glycerin. Using a hand mixer, beat at high speed for 1 minute.

5. Pour or spoon mixture into glass jars. Let cool.

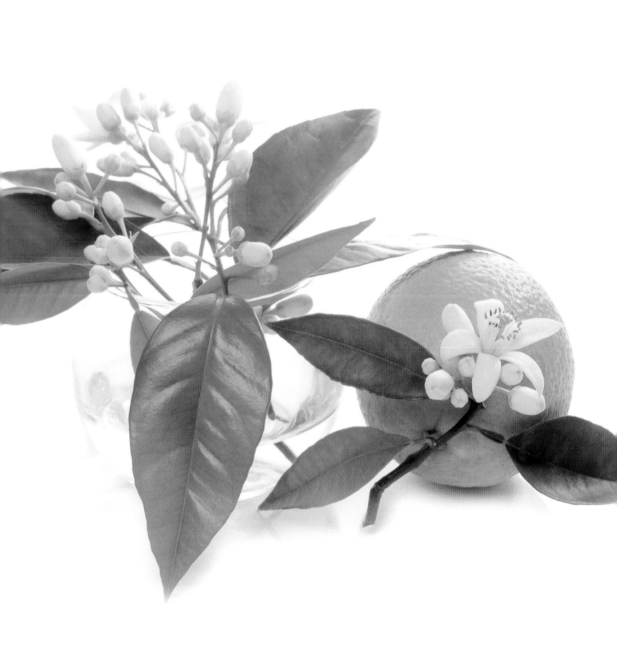

Baobab and Cedar Moisturizing Body Cream

This cream is recommended for skin that is dry and prone to flaking. It's excellent for protecting skin from winter weather and makes every skin tone, from dark to fair, look radiant.

Best for: Dry to very dry skin

Tips: Pure shea butter comes in chunks, like cocoa butter, at cosmetic-supply stores. Break or chop it up before adding it to the saucepan so that it melts quickly and easily.

Liquid glycerin is a moisturizing ingredient often included in cosmetics, soaps, shampoos and creams. You'll find small bottles of it at drugstores, but cosmetic-supply stores sell larger bulk amounts.

1 oz	baobab oil	30 g
0.4 oz	Lanette wax (see box, page 15)	12 g
0.35 oz	shea butter (see tips, at left)	10 g
12.3 oz	mineral water	350 g
4	pinches citric acid powder (see box, page 27)	4
4	pinches ascorbic acid powder	4
0.35 oz	liquid glycerin (see tips, at left)	10 g
15	drops cedar essential oil	15

1. Combine baobab oil, Lanette wax and shea butter in a saucepan. Heat over low heat just until ingredients are completely melted. Remove from heat and keep warm.

2. Pour mineral water into a separate saucepan. Heat until lukewarm. Using a wooden spoon, stir in citric acid and ascorbic acid until dissolved.

3. Stir mineral water mixture into oil mixture. Using a hand mixer, beat at low speed for 1 to 2 minutes. Let stand for 10 minutes.

4. Stir in glycerin and cedar essential oil. Using a hand mixer, beat at high speed for 1 minute.

5. Pour or spoon mixture into glass jars. Let cool.

Baobab Eye Cream

This eye cream is especially good for young skin. The delicate tissue under the eyes absorbs this non-greasy formula with ease.

Best for: All skin types

Tip: Rose water is often used in Middle Eastern and Mediterranean cooking. Look for it in Middle Eastern grocery stores and some well-stocked supermarkets.

Note: Exact measurements are important when you're making skin- and hair-care products. Turn to page 17 for how-tos.

0.35 oz	baobab oil	10 g
0.07 oz	Lanette wax (see box, page 15)	2 g
1 oz	rose water (see tip, at left)	30 g
1	pinch ascorbic acid powder (see box, page 27)	1
2	drops geranium essential oil	2

1. Combine baobab oil and Lanette wax in a saucepan. Heat over low heat just until ingredients are completely melted. Remove from heat and keep warm.

2. Pour rose water into a separate saucepan. Heat until lukewarm. Using a wooden spoon, stir in ascorbic acid until dissolved.

3. Stir rose water mixture into oil mixture. Using a hand mixer, beat at low speed for 1 to 2 minutes. Let stand for 10 minutes.

4. Stir in geranium essential oil. Using a hand mixer, beat at high speed for 1 minute.

5. Pour or spoon mixture into glass jars. Let cool.

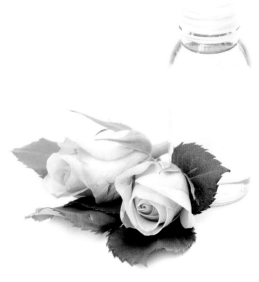

Baobab Sunscreen

This protective sunscreen is ideal for people who tan easily, but it doesn't offer enough protection for people with fair skin. In all cases, watch the time and limit your sun exposure as much as you can.

Best for: Skin that tans easily

Tip: Look for 100% pure beeswax that has been minimally processed. It is often sold in bulk, in chunks; if the recipe calls for a large amount, grate the wax so it will melt quickly and smoothly. Alternatively, you can buy beeswax pearls, which are easy to measure and melt quickly.

Note: Exact measurements are important when you're making skin- and hair-care products. Turn to page 17 for how-tos.

0.5 oz	avocado oil (see tip, below)	15 g
0.5 oz	walnut oil	15 g
0.4 oz	Lanette wax (see box, page 15)	12 g
0.35 oz	baobab oil	10 g
0.15 oz	beeswax (see tip, at left)	4 g
10.8 oz	orange flower water	305 g
4	pinches citric acid powder (see box, page 27)	4
4	pinches ascorbic acid powder	4
0.18 oz	carrot seed essential oil	5 g

1. Combine avocado oil, walnut oil, Lanette wax, baobab oil and beeswax in a saucepan. Heat over low heat just until ingredients are completely melted. Remove from heat and keep warm.

2. Pour orange flower water into a separate saucepan. Heat until lukewarm. Using a wooden spoon, stir in citric acid and ascorbic acid until dissolved.

3. Stir orange flower water mixture into oil mixture. Using a hand mixer, beat at low speed for 1 to 2 minutes. Let stand for 10 minutes.

4. Stir in carrot seed essential oil. Using a hand mixer, beat at high speed for 1 minute.

5. Pour or spoon mixture into glass jars. Let cool.

Tip: Avocado oil can vary from pale golden to dark green, so your finished cream might be a different color than shown in the photo (opposite).

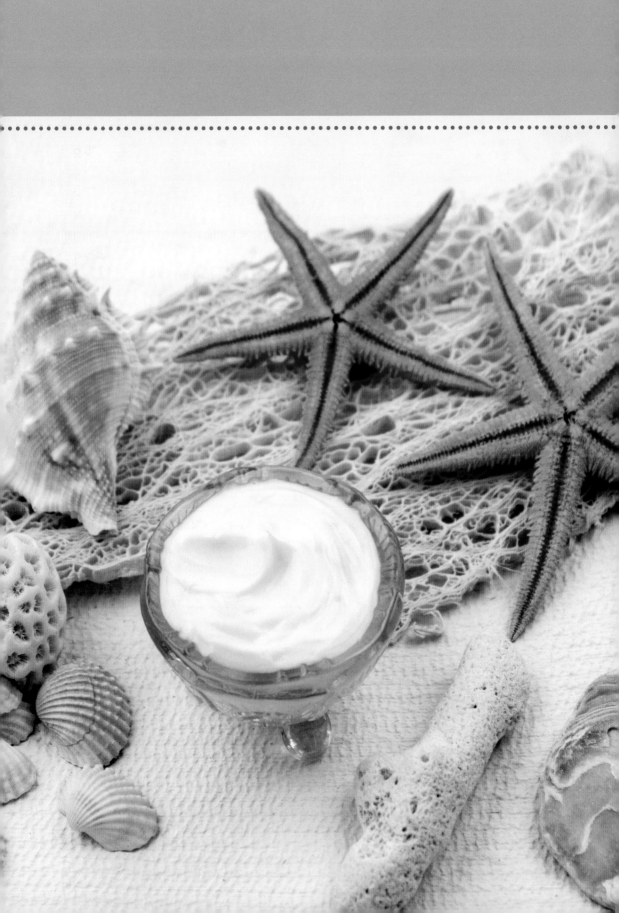

Baobab and Ylang-Ylang Massage Oil

It doesn't get simpler than this recipe. The gentle perfume of ylang-ylang adds an exotic touch.

Best for: All skin types

Note: Exact measurements are important when you're making skin- and hair-care products. Turn to page 17 for how-tos.

| 0.7 oz | baobab oil | 20 g |
| 10 | drops ylang-ylang essential oil | 10 |

1. Pour baobab oil and ylang-ylang essential oil into a small glass bottle. Seal tightly.
2. Shake to combine.

Tip: Use this oil to give yourself (or someone you love) a soothing hand massage. Spread a generous amount over the hands and begin to massage, kneading the fleshy parts of the palms and pulling on each finger as you rub from knuckle to tip.

Baobab Moisturizing Facial Oil

Facial moisturizer doesn't always need to be a cream. Oils like this can be very effective and rejuvenating.

Best for: Normal or combination skin

1 oz	baobab oil	30 g
5	drops cedar essential oil	5
6	drops sandalwood essential oil	6

1. Pour baobab oil, and cedar and sandalwood essential oils into a small glass bottle. Seal tightly.
2. Shake to combine.

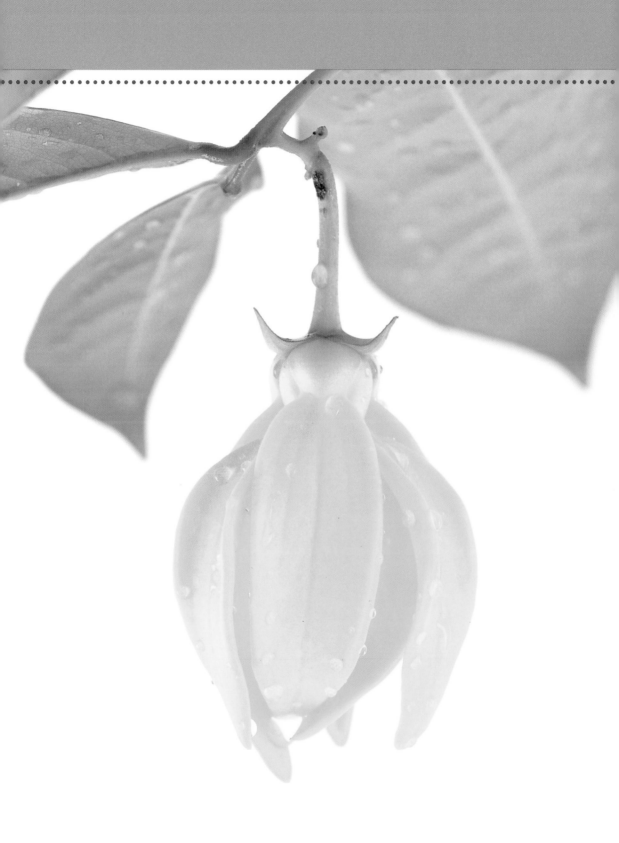

Baobab Nourishing Facial Oil

Rosewood essential oil gives this nutrient-rich formula a subtle scent, with both woody and floral notes.

Best for: Normal or combination skin

1 oz	baobab oil	30 g
5	drops rosewood essential oil (see tip, below)	5

1. Pour baobab oil and rosewood essential oil into a small glass bottle. Seal tightly.

2. Shake to combine.

Tip: The evergreen rosewood tree is an endangered and protected species in its native Brazil, so make sure you buy sustainably sourced rosewood essential oil. If you don't see any information on the label, ask the producer to disclose the source of the oil.

Baobab and Chamomile Facial Oil

Chamomile essential oil soothes dry skin, and adds a delicate aroma to this moisturizing treatment.

Best for: Dry, flaky skin

Note: Exact measurements are important when you're making skin- and hair-care products. Turn to page 17 for how-tos.

0.5 oz	baobab oil	15 g
0.5 oz	St. John's wort oil	15 g
5	drops chamomile essential oil (see tip, below)	5

1. Pour baobab oil, St. John's wort oil and chamomile essential oil into a small glass bottle. Seal tightly.

2. Shake to combine.

Tip: You'll often find two types of chamomile essential oil at cosmetic-supply stores: German and Roman. They come from different strains of the chamomile plant, but both are soothing additions to homemade skin- and hair-care products.

Baobab Body Oil

If you're in need of a wonderful-smelling, totally soothing body oil, look no further. The combination of almond and petitgrain oils is divine.

Best for: All skin types

Tip: Petitgrain essential oil is made from the leaves and twigs of the bitter orange tree. It has a beautiful scent that is different from the scents of orange and neroli essential oils, which are made from other parts of the tree. Petitgrain essential oil is often added to perfumes.

Note: Exact measurements are important when you're making skin- and hair-care products. Turn to page 17 for how-tos.

5.3 oz	baobab oil	150 g
0.9 oz	sweet almond oil	25 g
0.1 oz	petitgrain essential oil (see tip, at left)	3 g

1. Pour baobab oil, sweet almond oil and petitgrain essential oil into a small glass bottle. Seal tightly.

2. Shake to combine.

Baobab Oil on Its Own

Baobab oil can be used alone, without any additions, to moisturize and nourish the skin. It is good for both the face and the rest of the body. Pour a small amount of the oil into the palm of your hand, then warm it by rubbing your hands together vigorously. Apply the oil to your skin and massage gently. For chapped lips, place a drop of baobab oil on your fingertip and spread it gently across your lips.

Baobab Hair Repair Oil

Cutting off split ends is the only way to totally get rid of them, but this healing oil helps smooth them and prevent them from starting in the first place.

Best for: Damaged or damage-prone hair

Note: Exact measurements are important when you're making skin- and hair-care products. Turn to page 17 for how-tos.

0.35 oz	pure vitamin E (see tips, below)	10 g
0.18 oz	baobab oil	5 g

1. Pour vitamin E and baobab oil into a small glass bottle. Seal tightly.
2. Shake to combine.

Tips: Look for pure vitamin E in liquid form at cosmetic-supply stores. It's also easy to find online. You can also use the contents of vitamin E capsules purchased at the pharmacy.

To apply, massage the oil into the ends of your hair with your fingertips 1 hour before washing. If your hair is very dry and damaged, apply a small amount just before blow-drying.

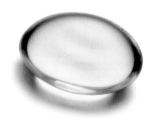

Baobab Exfoliating Scrub

This excellent exfoliant removes dead skin cells, gently rubs away calluses and heals small cracks, especially in the heels, that are caused by dry skin. Baobab oil nourishes the skin as you scrub.

Best for: Rough skin, especially on the elbows, knees and heels

Note: Exact measurements are important when you're making skin- and hair-care products. Turn to page 17 for how-tos.

1.8 oz	fine sea salt	50 g
1.4 oz	baobab oil	40 g
5	drops cedar essential oil	5

1. Combine sea salt, baobab oil and cedar essential oil in a bowl.
2. Using a wooden spoon, stir until ingredients are well combined. Use immediately.

Tip: To apply, place a little bit of the scrub (about 1 tsp/5 mL) in the palm of your hand and rub in gentle circles over the area to be treated.

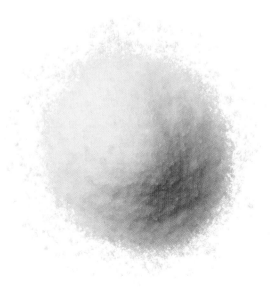

Baobab and Chamomile Shampoo

This shampoo is recommended for everyday dry hair. It is also excellent to take along on a beach vacation, when hair needs extra moisturizing after exposure to sun and sand.

Best for: Dry to very dry hair

Tips: Coco betaine (short for cocamido-propyl betaine) is a surfactant made from coconut oil and gives shampoos their cleaning power and lather. It's easy to find at cosmetic-supply stores.

You'll often find two types of chamomile essential oil at cosmetic-supply stores: German and Roman. They come from different strains of the chamomile plant, but both are soothing additions to homemade skin- and hair-care products.

2 tbsp	fresh or dried chamomile flowers	30 mL
7.2 oz	mineral water	205 g
5.3 oz	coco betaine (see tips, at left)	150 g
0.35 oz	baobab oil	10 g
20	drops chamomile essential oil (see tips, at left)	20

1. Place chamomile flowers in a heatproof bowl. In a saucepan, bring mineral water to a boil. Pour boiling mineral water over chamomile flowers. Cover and let steep for 10 minutes.

2. Using a fine-mesh sieve lined with cheesecloth, strain the infusion into a clean bowl. Let cool completely.

3. Pour chamomile infusion, coco betaine, baobab oil and chamomile essential oil into a bottle. Shake gently to combine.

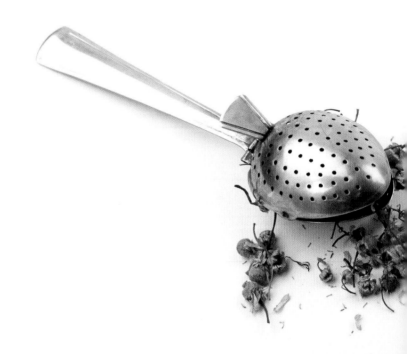

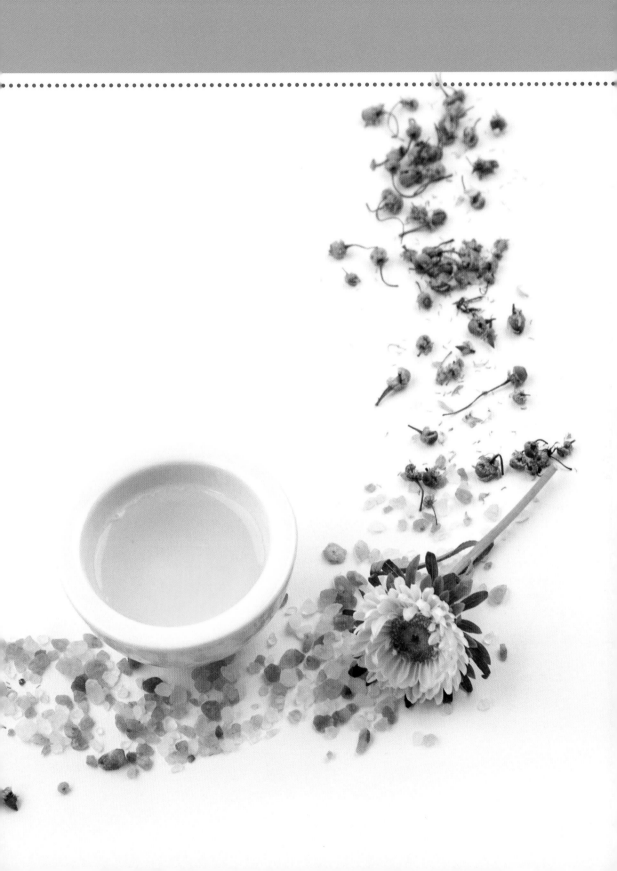

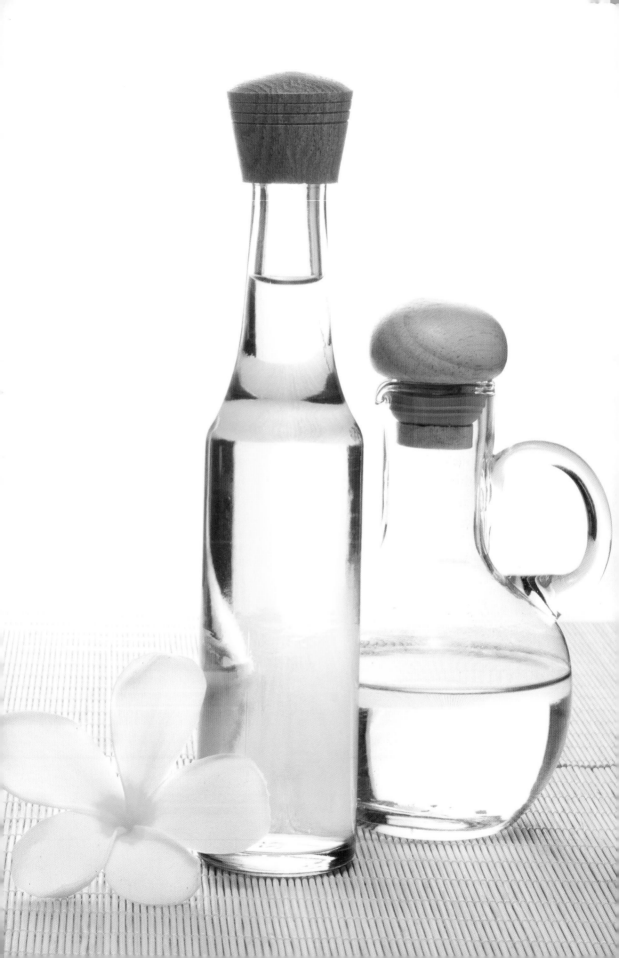

Monoï Oil

Monoï oil is suitable for all skin types.
The main benefit it offers is its powerful
skin-firming ability.

The origins of monoï oil date back some 2,000 years. The indigenous Polynesian Maori people of Aotearoa (better known as New Zealand in English) used it for medicinal, cosmetic and religious purposes. It was applied to babies' skin to keep them from dehydrating in hot weather and to protect them in cold weather. The bodies of the dead were embalmed and perfumed with monoï. Maori sailors also traditionally used it to protect their skin from salt water and cold during long canoe expeditions. Today, many Polynesian divers still rub monoï oil all over their bodies before a long plunge in the ocean.

Monoï oil is the great beauty secret of Tahitian women. It is also the main oil used in Polynesian massage, because it has moisturizing, soothing and nourishing properties for both skin and hair. In the warm summer months, it can help protect hair from the damaging effects of sun and sea. It also helps reduce dandruff, and even makes tans last longer.

If you're ever lucky enough to have access to fresh tiare flowers — the quintessential blooms of Polynesia — you can make this fragrant, delicate oil. Simply marinate the flowers in coconut oil for several days, and you will have a homemade version of this prized oil laced with the unmistakable scent of the flowers.

Monoï Moisturizing Face Cream

Smooth, silky and gorgeously scented, this cream works on all types of skin, and for people of all ages.

Best for: All skin types

Tip: Rose water is often used in Middle Eastern and Mediterranean cooking. Look for it in Middle Eastern grocery stores and some well-stocked supermarkets.

Note: Exact measurements are important when you're making skin- and hair-care products. Turn to page 17 for how-tos.

0.7 oz	monoï oil	20 g
0.2 oz	Lanette wax (see box, page 15)	6 g
0.18 oz	cocoa butter (see tips, below)	5 g
6 oz	rose water (see tip, at left)	170 g
2	pinches citric acid powder (see box, page 27)	2
2	pinches ascorbic acid powder	2
10	drops geranium essential oil	10

1. Combine monoï oil, Lanette wax and cocoa butter in a saucepan. Heat over low heat just until ingredients are completely melted. Remove from heat and keep warm.

2. Pour rose water into a separate saucepan. Heat until lukewarm. Using a wooden spoon, stir in citric acid and ascorbic acid until dissolved.

3. Stir rose water mixture into oil mixture. Using a hand mixer, beat at low speed for 1 to 2 minutes. Let stand for 10 minutes.

4. Stir in geranium essential oil. Using a hand mixer, beat at high speed for 1 minute.

5. Pour or spoon mixture into glass jars. Let cool.

Tips: Look for chunks or blocks of pure cocoa butter at cosmetic-supply stores. If you're using a large amount in a recipe, chop it up before adding it to the saucepan so it will melt more quickly.

Choose 100% natural cocoa butter to make the recipes in this book. It can vary in color from pale cream to brownish yellow.

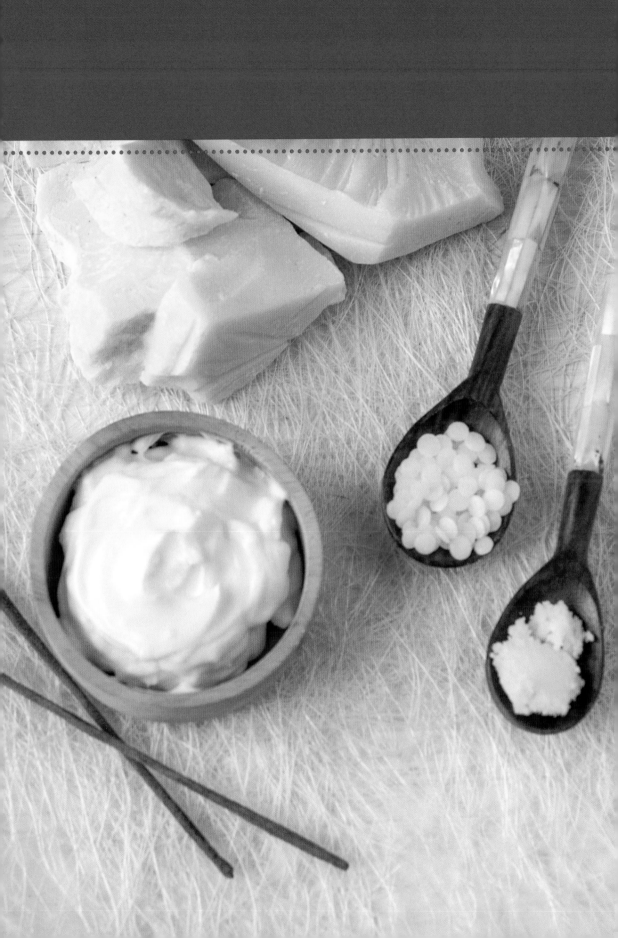

Monoï Firming Body Cream

Scented with a blend of essential oils, this cream feels and smells luxurious. It will quench your skin's thirst beautifully.

Best for: Sagging, dehydrated skin

Tips: Pure shea butter comes in chunks, like cocoa butter, at cosmetic-supply stores. Break or chop it up before adding it to the saucepan so that it melts quickly and easily.

The essential oils you use for skin- and hair-care products must be 100% pure. Don't use synthetic scents or oils, or essences used in fragrance burners or lamp rings.

Note: Exact measurements are important when you're making skin- and hair-care products. Turn to page 17 for how-tos.

1.4 oz	monoï oil	40 g
0.4 oz	Lanette wax (see box, page 15)	12 g
0.35 oz	hazelnut oil	10 g
0.35 oz	shea butter (see tips, at left)	10 g
11.3 oz	mineral water	320 g
4	pinches citric acid powder (see box, page 27)	4
4	pinches ascorbic acid powder	4
0.7 oz	liquid glycerin	20 g
10	drops cypress essential oil (see tips, at left)	10
10	drops geranium essential oil	10
10	drops patchouli essential oil	10
10	drops frankincense essential oil	10
10	drops lemongrass essential oil	10

1. Combine monoï oil, Lanette wax, hazelnut oil and shea butter in a saucepan. Heat over low heat just until ingredients are completely melted. Remove from heat and keep warm.

2. Pour mineral water into a separate saucepan. Heat until lukewarm. Using a wooden spoon, stir in citric acid and ascorbic acid until dissolved.

3. Stir mineral water mixture into oil mixture. Using a hand mixer, beat at low speed for 1 to 2 minutes. Let stand for 10 minutes.

4. Stir in glycerin, and cypress, geranium, patchouli, frankincense and lemongrass essential oils. Using a hand mixer, beat at high speed for 1 minute.

5. Pour or spoon mixture into glass jars. Let cool.

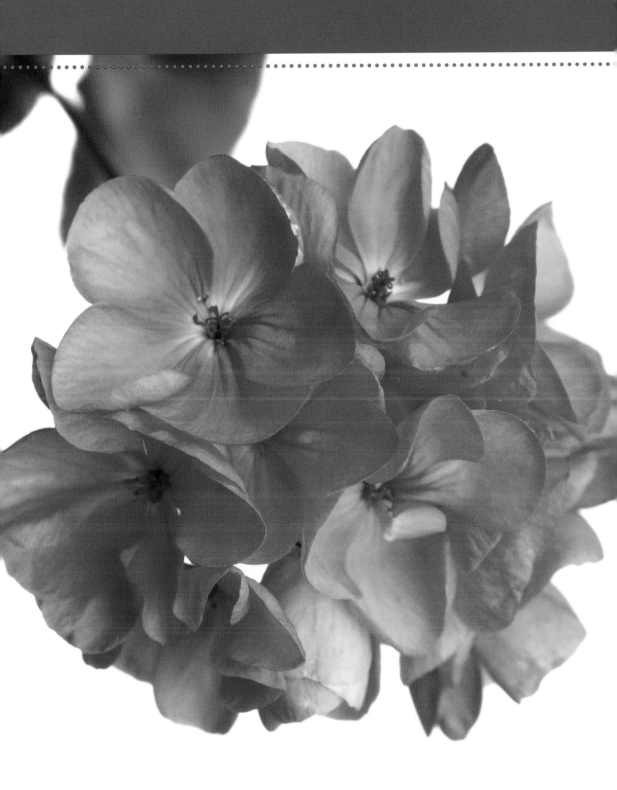

Monoï and Orange Moisturizing Body Cream

When you need an all-purpose body cream, this is an excellent choice. Its orange scent will wake you up as you smooth it on.

• ❀ •

Best for: All skin types

Tips: Orange flower water is also called orange blossom water. It's easy to find in Middle Eastern grocery stores and some well-stocked supermarkets, where it's sold for use in cooking.

Neroli essential oil is distilled from the flowers of the orange tree. It is a comparatively expensive essential oil, but its fragrance is absolutely heavenly and worth the price. You may also see it under the name orange flower essential oil.

1.4 oz	monoï oil	40 g
0.4 oz	Lanette wax (see box, page 15)	12 g
0.35 oz	cocoa butter	10 g
11.6 oz	orange flower water (see tips, at left)	330 g
4	pinches citric acid powder (see box, page 27)	4
4	pinches ascorbic acid powder	4
5	drops neroli essential oil (see tips, at left)	5

1. Combine monoï oil, Lanette wax and cocoa butter in a saucepan. Heat over low heat just until ingredients are completely melted. Remove from heat and keep warm.

2. Pour orange flower water into a separate saucepan. Heat until lukewarm. Using a wooden spoon, stir in citric acid and ascorbic acid until dissolved.

3. Stir orange flower water mixture into oil mixture. Using a hand mixer, beat at low speed for 1 to 2 minutes. Let stand for 10 minutes.

4. Stir in neroli essential oil. Using a hand mixer, beat at high speed for 1 minute.

5. Pour or spoon mixture into glass jars. Let cool.

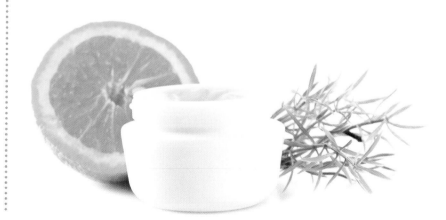

Monoï Tan Extender Cream

Sure, you need to be careful of sun exposure. But why not preserve the tan you have for as long as you can? This cream will help you maintain your glow past the end of summer.

Best for: Skin that tans easily

Tip: Look for 100% pure beeswax that has been minimally processed. It is often sold in bulk, in chunks; if the recipe calls for a large amount, grate the wax so it will melt quickly and smoothly. Alternatively, you can buy beeswax pearls, which are easy to measure and melt quickly.

Note: Exact measurements are important when you're making skin- and hair-care products. Turn to page 17 for how-tos.

0.35 oz	monoï oil	10 g
0.18 oz	avocado oil	5 g
0.1 oz	beeswax (see tip, at left)	3 g
6.2 oz	mineral water	175 g
2	pinches citric acid powder (see box, page 27)	2
2	pinches ascorbic acid powder	2
0.18 oz	carrot seed essential oil	5 g

1. Combine monoï oil, avocado oil and beeswax in a saucepan. Heat over low heat just until ingredients are completely melted. Remove from heat and keep warm.

2. Pour mineral water into a separate saucepan. Heat until lukewarm. Using a wooden spoon, stir in citric acid and ascorbic acid until dissolved.

3. Stir mineral water mixture into oil mixture. Using a hand mixer, beat at low speed for 1 to 2 minutes. Let stand for 10 minutes.

4. Stir in carrot seed essential oil. Using a hand mixer, beat at high speed for 1 minute.

5. Pour or spoon mixture into glass jars. Let cool.

Monoï Oil Repairs Tired Summer Hair

It is a good idea to nourish your hair after long exposure to sun, salt water or chlorinated pool water. If you have dry to very dry hair, place a few drops of monoï oil on your fingertips and massage it all through your hair, especially the ends. Then wash as usual. You'll love the shiny, well-nourished results.

Monoï Hand Cream

This cream is ideal for use any time of day. The skin absorbs it quickly, and it doesn't leave your hands feeling greasy.

Best for: Normal to dry hands

Tips: Look for chunks or blocks of pure cocoa butter at cosmetic-supply stores. If you're using a large amount in a recipe, chop it up before adding it to the saucepan so it will melt more quickly.

Liquid glycerin is a moisturizing ingredient often included in cosmetics, soaps, shampoos and creams. You'll find small bottles of it at drugstores, but cosmetic-supply stores sell larger bulk amounts.

Note: Exact measurements are important when you're making skin- and hair-care products. Turn to page 17 for how-tos.

0.5 oz	monoï oil	15 g
0.2 oz	Lanette wax (see box, page 15)	6 g
0.18 oz	cocoa butter (see tips, at left)	5 g
5.6 oz	witch hazel	160 g
2	pinches citric acid powder (see box, page 27)	2
2	pinches ascorbic acid powder	2
0.35 oz	liquid glycerin (see tips, at left)	10 g

1. Combine monoï oil, Lanette wax and cocoa butter in a saucepan. Heat over low heat just until ingredients are completely melted. Remove from heat and keep warm.

2. Pour witch hazel into a separate saucepan. Heat until lukewarm. Using a wooden spoon, stir in citric acid and ascorbic acid until dissolved.

3. Stir witch hazel mixture into oil mixture. Using a hand mixer, beat at low speed for 1 to 2 minutes. Let stand for 10 minutes.

4. Stir in glycerin. Using a hand mixer, beat at high speed for 1 minute.

5. Pour or spoon mixture into glass jars. Let cool.

Monoï Oil for Massages

Monoï oil is an exceptional massage oil on its own. It is highly moisturizing and easily absorbed, and doesn't leave the skin feeling greasy. For a relaxing massage, warm the oil slightly; it will bathe the senses with its gentle flower scent and smooth sensation on the skin. It can be mixed with other base oils and even essential oils for therapeutic use.

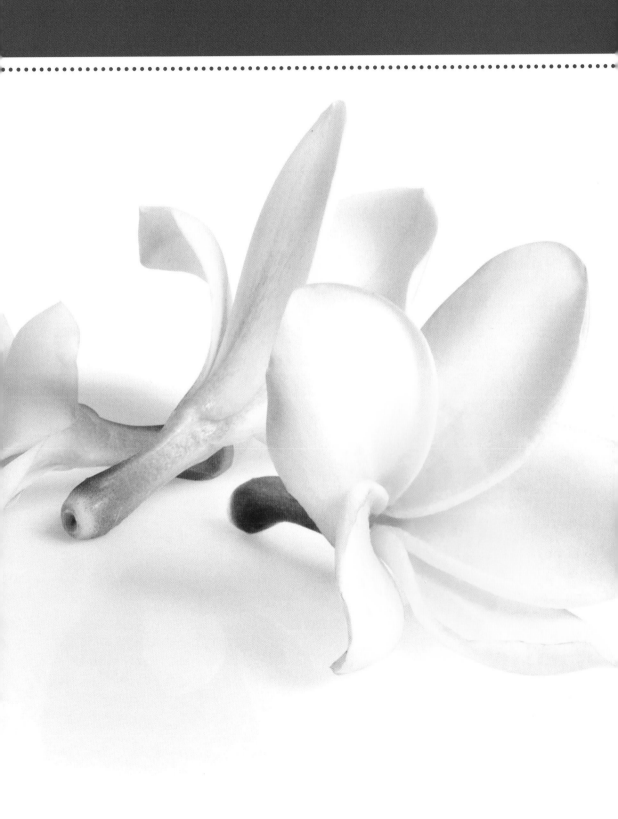

Monoï Nourishing Skin Oil

This refreshing oil works all over the body and is nice for the face, as well. It firms and moisturizes at the same time.

Best for: Loose, sagging skin

Tip: To apply the oil, place a small amount in the palm of your hand, then rub your hands together to warm it. Spread it over the face or body, wherever your skin needs firming.

Note: Exact measurements are important when you're making skin- and hair-care products. Turn to page 17 for how-tos.

0.35 oz	monoï oil	10 g
0.18 oz	St. John's wort oil	5 g
10	drops lemongrass essential oil	10
5	drops patchouli essential oil	5
5	drops lemon essential oil	5

1. Pour monoï oil, St. John's wort oil, and lemongrass, patchouli and lemon essential oils into a small glass bottle. Seal tightly.

2. Shake to combine.

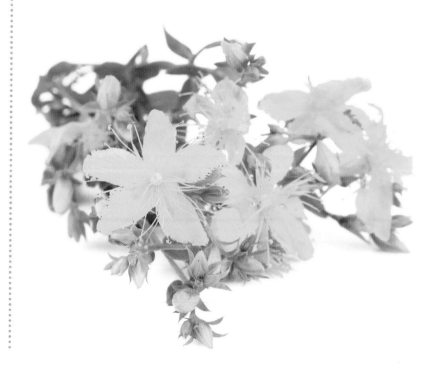

Monoï and Sage Dandruff Shampoo

The scent of Spanish sage makes this natural dandruff fighter smell so much better than commercial versions made with chemicals.

Best for: Scalps with occasional or chronic dandruff

Note: Exact measurements are important when you're making skin- and hair-care products. Turn to page 17 for how-tos.

3.5 oz	mineral water	100 g
3.5 oz	coco betaine (see tips, below)	100 g
0.25 oz	cider vinegar	7 g
0.18 oz	monoï oil	5 g
30	drops Spanish sage essential oil (see tips, below)	30

1. Pour mineral water, coco betaine, cider vinegar, monoï oil and Spanish sage essential oil into a bottle.

2. Shake gently to combine.

Tips: Coco betaine (short for cocamidopropyl betaine) is a surfactant made from coconut oil and gives shampoos their cleaning power and lather. It's easy to find at cosmetic-supply stores.

Spanish sage *(Salvia lavandulifolia)* is one of many different types of sage, each of which has unique therapeutic properties. This variety is excellent at curbing dandruff, so make sure that's the base of the essential oil you add to this formula.

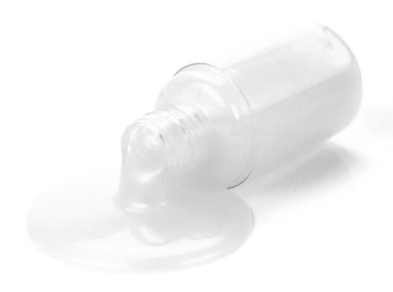

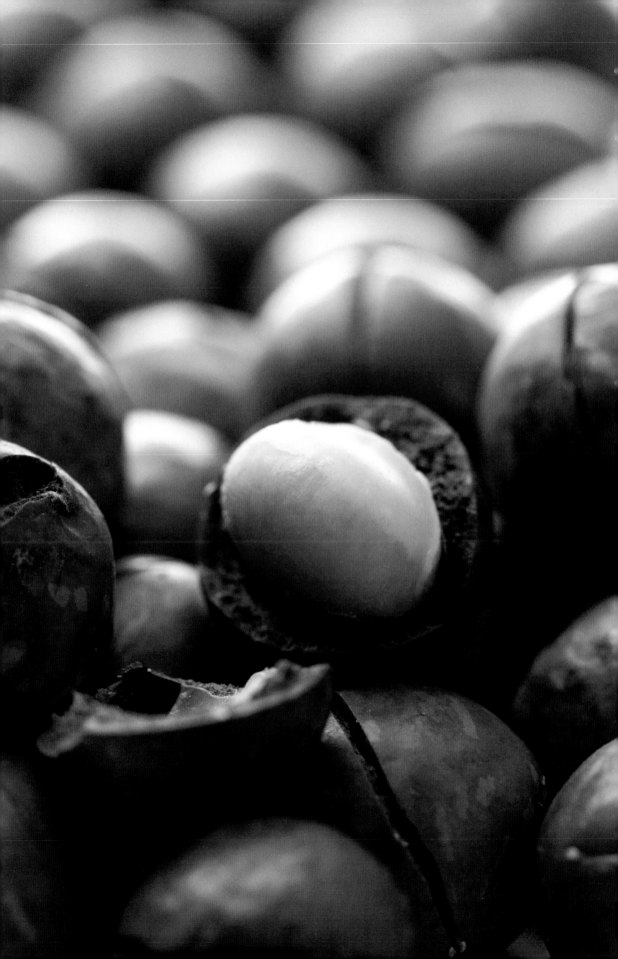

Macadamia Oil

Macadamia oil readily penetrates the skin and serves as an excellent vehicle for the absorption of essential oils.

This oil is extracted from the macadamia nut *(Macadamia integrifolia),* which is native to the forests of eastern Australia. In the late 19th century, this nut was introduced to Hawaii, where it flourished. Hawaii remains one of the world's leading macadamia-producing regions.

It is the only vegetable oil that contains large amounts of palmitoleic acid, a monounsaturated fatty acid. In fact, it is the oil that is richest in monounsaturated fatty acids (they make up about 80% of its fat content). Macadamia oil has been used for thousands of years by the Australian Aborigines, and is very popular in Australian haute cuisine because of its delicate, slightly sweet flavor.

Macadamia oil is light, which makes it suitable for many skin-care formulas. It is rich in oleic and linoleic acids and sterols (especially avenasterol). It keeps the skin healthy and glowing, and also has soothing and calming properties. It is suitable for devitalized and sagging skin, because it helps restore firmness and elasticity. It is a noncomedogenic oil, which means that it helps the skin retain its natural moisture without clogging pores. Its high vitamin E content helps protect against sun damage and free radicals.

Macadamia Face Cream for Sensitive Skin

This cream is soothing and extremely gentle for skin of all ages. Rose water and lavender essential oil give it a timeless, relaxing scent.

Best for: Sensitive skin, especially for children and seniors

Tips: Look for chunks or blocks of pure cocoa butter at cosmetic-supply stores. If you're using a large amount in a recipe, chop it up before adding it to the saucepan so it will melt more quickly.

Rose water is often used in Middle Eastern and Mediterranean cooking. Look for it in Middle Eastern grocery stores and some well-stocked supermarkets.

Note: Exact measurements are important when you're making skin- and hair-care products. Turn to page 17 for how-tos.

0.7 oz	macadamia oil	20 g
0.2 oz	Lanette wax (see box, page 15)	6 g
0.18 oz	cocoa butter (see tips, at left)	5 g
5.8 oz	rose water (see tips, at left)	165 g
2	pinches citric acid powder (see box, page 27)	2
2	pinches ascorbic acid powder	2
6	drops lavender essential oil	6

1. Combine macadamia oil, Lanette wax and cocoa butter in a saucepan. Heat over low heat just until ingredients are completely melted. Remove from heat and keep warm.

2. Pour rose water into a separate saucepan. Heat until lukewarm. Using a wooden spoon, stir in citric acid and ascorbic acid until dissolved.

3. Stir rose water mixture into oil mixture. Using a hand mixer, beat at low speed for 1 to 2 minutes. Let stand for 10 minutes.

4. Stir in lavender essential oil. Using a hand mixer, beat at high speed for 1 minute.

5. Pour or spoon mixture into glass jars. Let cool.

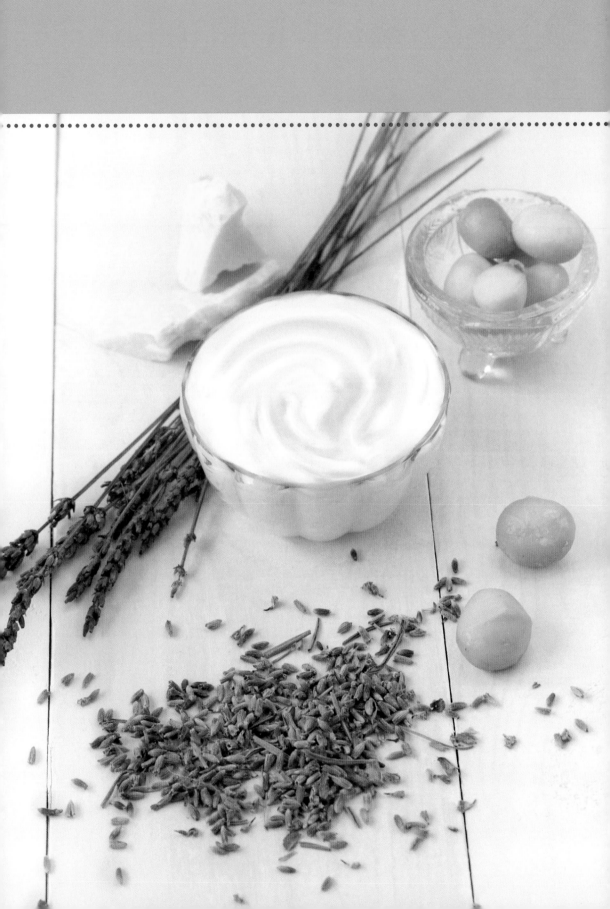

Macadamia Moisturizing Body Cream

When you use this cream, you'll quickly see improvement. It's especially effective for treating the fragile skin of the elderly.

Best for: Sensitive skin, especially for children and seniors

Tips: Pure shea butter comes in chunks, like cocoa butter, and is sold at cosmetic-supply stores. Break or chop it up before adding it to the saucepan so that it melts quickly and easily.

Orange flower water is also called orange blossom water. It's easy to find in Middle Eastern grocery stores and some well-stocked supermarkets, where it's sold for use in cooking.

Note: Exact measurements are important when you're making skin- and hair-care products. Turn to page 17 for how-tos.

1 oz	macadamia oil	30 g
0.4 oz	Lanette wax (see box, page 15)	12 g
0.2 oz	shea butter (see tips, at left)	6 g
11.6 oz	orange flower water (see tips, at left)	330 g
4	pinches citric acid powder (see box, page 27)	4
4	pinches ascorbic acid powder	4
0.7 oz	liquid glycerin	20 g
20	drops lavender essential oil	20

1. Combine macadamia oil, Lanette wax and shea butter in a saucepan. Heat over low heat just until ingredients are completely melted. Remove from heat and keep warm.

2. Pour orange flower water into a separate saucepan. Heat until lukewarm. Using a wooden spoon, stir in citric acid and ascorbic acid until dissolved.

3. Stir orange flower water mixture into oil mixture. Using a hand mixer, beat at low speed for 1 to 2 minutes. Let stand for 10 minutes.

4. Stir in glycerin and lavender essential oil. Using a hand mixer, beat at high speed for 1 minute.

5. Pour or spoon mixture into glass jars. Let cool.

Macadamia and Collagen Nourishing Face Cream

This is an intense restoring cream for withered, heavily damaged skin. It is recommended for women experiencing perimenopause and those in the later stages of life.

Best for: Sagging, devitalized skin

Tips: Soluble collagen is a moisturizing ingredient that is often added to cosmetics. It comes in powder form at cosmetic-supply stores.

The essential oils you use for skin- and hair-care products must be 100% pure. Don't use synthetic scents or oils, or essences used in fragrance burners or lamp rings.

Note: Exact measurements are important when you're making skin- and hair-care products. Turn to page 17 for how-tos.

1 oz	macadamia oil	30 g
0.35 oz	sesame oil	10 g
0.28 oz	St. John's wort oil	8 g
0.2 oz	Lanette wax (see box, page 15)	6 g
0.18 oz	cocoa butter	5 g
3.9 oz	witch hazel	110 g
2	pinches citric acid powder (see box, page 27)	2
2	pinches ascorbic acid powder	2
1 oz	soluble collagen (see tips, at left)	30 g
20	drops myrrh essential oil (see tips, at left)	20

1. Combine macadamia oil, sesame oil, St. John's wort oil, Lanette wax and cocoa butter in a saucepan. Heat over low heat just until ingredients are completely melted. Remove from heat and keep warm.

2. Pour witch hazel into a separate saucepan. Heat until lukewarm. Using a wooden spoon, stir in citric acid and ascorbic acid until dissolved.

3. Stir witch hazel mixture into oil mixture. Using a hand mixer, beat at low speed for 1 to 2 minutes. Let stand for 10 minutes.

4. Stir in collagen and myrrh essential oil. Using a hand mixer, beat at high speed for 1 minute.

5. Pour or spoon mixture into glass jars. Let cool.

Vitamin-Rich Macadamia Moisturizing Face Cream

This cream is good for women who are experiencing menopause, a time when the skin loses elasticity and tone.

Best for: Sagging, devitalized skin

Tip: Look for pure vitamins A and E in liquid form at cosmetic-supply stores. They're also easy to buy online.

Note: Exact measurements are important when you're making skin- and hair-care products. Turn to page 17 for how-tos.

0.35 oz	macadamia oil	10 g
0.35 oz	sesame oil	10 g
0.2 oz	Lanette wax (see box, page 15)	6 g
0.18 oz	cocoa butter	5 g
5.6 oz	witch hazel	160 g
2	pinches citric acid powder (see box, page 27)	2
2	pinches ascorbic acid powder	2
0.15 oz	pure vitamin A (see tip, at left)	4 g
0.07 oz	pure vitamin E	2 g
15	drops cedar essential oil	15

1. Combine macadamia oil, sesame oil, Lanette wax and cocoa butter in a saucepan. Heat over low heat just until ingredients are completely melted. Remove from heat and keep warm.

2. Pour witch hazel into a separate saucepan. Heat until lukewarm. Using a wooden spoon, stir in citric acid and ascorbic acid until dissolved.

3. Stir witch hazel mixture into oil mixture. Using a hand mixer, beat at low speed for 1 to 2 minutes. Let stand for 10 minutes.

4. Stir in vitamins A and E, and cedar essential oil. Using a hand mixer, beat at high speed for 1 minute.

5. Pour or spoon mixture into glass jars. Let cool.

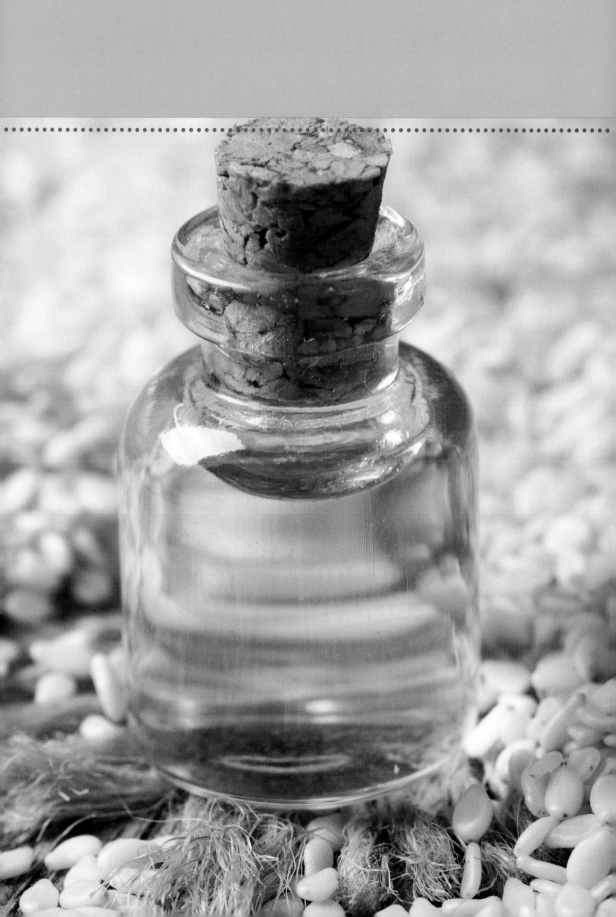

Macadamia Moisturizing Face Cream for Oily Skin

This emulsion is ideal for skin that tends to get oily and develop blackheads on the forehead, chin and sides of the nose.

Best for: Oily skin with blackheads

Tip: Rosemary is a wonderful herb for cooking and making body-care products. It grows easily and requires little care, so plant some in a pot or your garden and enjoy it all summer.

Note: Exact measurements are important when you're making skin- and hair-care products. Turn to page 17 for how-tos.

2 tbsp	fresh or dried rosemary (see tip, at left)	30 mL
6.3 oz	mineral water	180 g
2	pinches citric acid powder (see box, page 27)	2
2	pinches ascorbic acid powder	2
0.5 oz	macadamia oil	15 g
0.2 oz	Lanette wax (see box, page 15)	6 g
0.1 oz	cocoa butter	3 g
8	drops tea tree essential oil	8
3	drops lemon essential oil	3

1. Place rosemary in a heatproof bowl. In a saucepan, bring mineral water to a boil. Pour boiling mineral water over rosemary. Cover and let steep for 10 minutes.

2. Using a fine-mesh sieve lined with cheesecloth, strain the infusion into a clean bowl. Let cool until lukewarm. Using a wooden spoon, stir in citric acid and ascorbic acid until dissolved. Keep warm.

3. Combine macadamia oil, Lanette wax and cocoa butter in a separate saucepan. Heat over low heat just until ingredients are completely melted. Remove from heat.

4. Stir rosemary infusion mixture into oil mixture. Using a hand mixer, beat at low speed for 1 to 2 minutes. Let stand for 10 minutes.

5. Stir in tea tree and lemon essential oils. Using a hand mixer, beat at high speed for 1 minute.

6. Pour or spoon mixture into glass jars. Let cool.

Macadamia Skin Repairing Oil

For facial application, store this oil in a small glass jar and apply a small amount to the face using the fingertips. For the body, transfer the oil to a roll-on applicator. Roll it along the body, then spread the oil with the palms of your hands.

Best for: Sagging, devitalized and undernourished skin

Tips: Store essential oils in a cool, dark place. Light exposure can diminish their healing properties.

Go easy when applying this oil. If you use too much at once, it will be difficult for the skin to absorb it quickly.

Note: Exact measurements are important when you're making skin- and hair-care products. Turn to page 17 for how-tos.

4.4 oz	macadamia oil	125 g
0.7 oz	hazelnut oil	20 g
0.7 oz	jojoba oil	20 g
0.35 oz	sesame oil	10 g
25	drops sandalwood essential oil (see tips, at left)	25
25	drops cedar essential oil	25
25	drops lemongrass essential oil	25

1. Pour macadamia oil, hazelnut oil, jojoba oil, sesame oil, and sandalwood, cedar and lemongrass essential oils into a small glass bottle. Seal tightly.

2. Shake to combine.

Essential Oils Enhance Macadamia Oil for Massages

Macadamia oil helps essential oils penetrate the skin, making it one of the best massage oils. To make a custom-crafted formula that's perfect for you, start with 0.9 oz (25 g) macadamia oil. To it, add 5 drops of one of the following essential oils, depending on the type of massage you'd like:

- **Relaxing:** Frankincense, sandalwood or thyme
- **Energizing:** Nutmeg, fennel or bay laurel
- **Anti-stress:** Grapefruit, vetiver or basil

Macadamia and Cocoa Butter Lip Balm

In the winter, cold weather makes your lips cry out for relief. This balm is just what you need to soothe and protect them.

Best for: Dry, cracked lips

Note: Exact measurements are important when you're making skin- and hair-care products. Turn to page 17 for how-tos.

0.38 oz	cocoa butter	11 g
0.1 oz	beeswax (see tip, below)	3 g
0.04 oz	macadamia oil	1 g
4	drops mandarin essential oil	4

1. Combine cocoa butter and beeswax in a saucepan. Heat over low heat just until completely melted. (Do not let mixture begin to smoke.) Remove from heat.

2. Stir in macadamia oil and mandarin essential oil. Pour into a small glass jar. Let cool until solidified.

Tip: Look for 100% pure beeswax that has been minimally processed. It is often sold in bulk, in chunks; if the recipe calls for a large amount, grate the wax so it will melt quickly and smoothly. Alternatively, you can buy beeswax that has been formed into pearls, which are easy to measure and melt quickly. Beeswax is a natural product, so the color can vary quite a bit. You will find it in shades ranging from nearly white to rich yellow to brown. No matter what color the wax is, its skin-healing properties are the same.

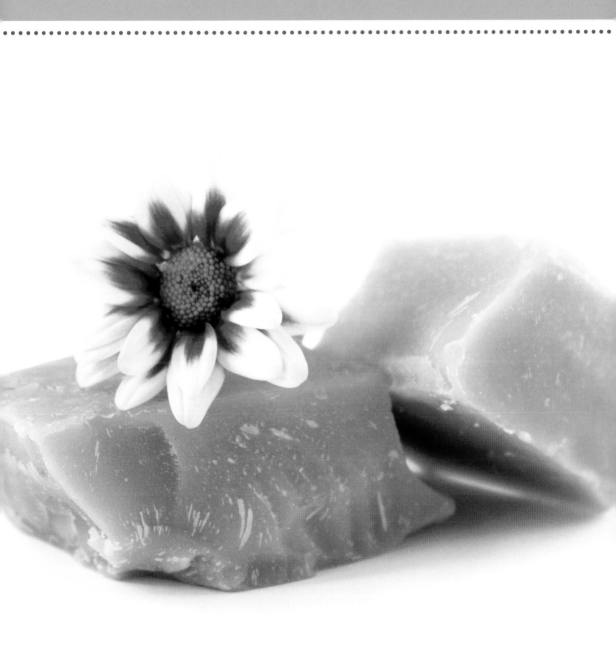

Macadamia and Green Clay Poultice

This old-fashioned mixture is just the thing to treat sore, aching muscles and banged-up skin. Combine it with rest and relaxation for a healing cure.

Best for: Sprains, bruises and strains

Note: Exact measurements are important when you're making skin- and hair-care products. Turn to page 17 for how-tos.

Caution: Do not use rosemary essential oil if you have epilepsy or high blood pressure.

0.5 oz	green clay (see tips, below)	15 g
0.38 oz	mineral water	11 g
0.15 oz	macadamia oil	4 g
10	drops ginger essential oil	10
10	drops rosemary essential oil (see caution, at left)	10
10	drops thyme essential oil	10

1. In a bowl, stir clay with mineral water until mixture is the consistency of mayonnaise.
2. Stir in macadamia oil, and ginger, rosemary and thyme essential oils until blended. Use immediately.

Tips: Green clay is often added to facial masks and treatments, and is thought to stimulate blood flow to injured areas and speed up the healing process. Look for it in powdered form at cosmetic-supply stores.

Apply the poultice to the area to be treated, then wrap the area with plastic wrap. Leave on for about 2 hours. Wipe off the poultice mixture with a damp sponge or towel.

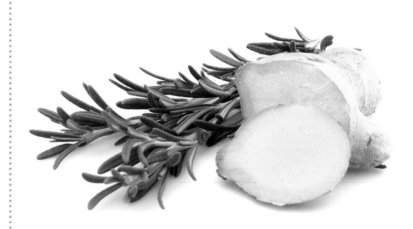

Macadamia and Sandalwood Body Scrub

Apply this lovely exfoliating scrub all over the body, including the face, and rub gently using a circular motion. Rinse it off with warm water and enjoy soft, fresh skin.

Best for: All skin types

Tip: Try this scrub at the end of a soothing bath for a special, pampering treat.

Note: Exact measurements are important when you're making skin- and hair-care products. Turn to page 17 for how-tos.

2.1 oz	fine sea salt	60 g
1.4 oz	macadamia oil	40 g
6	drops sandalwood or geranium essential oil	6

1. Combine sea salt, macadamia oil and sandalwood essential oil in a bowl.

2. Using a wooden spoon, stir well until ingredients are combined. Use immediately.

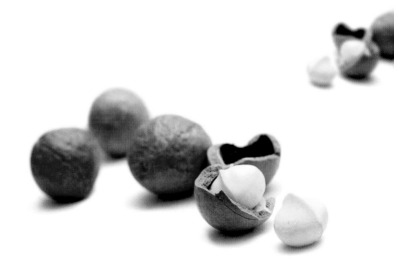

Macadamia Anti-Cellulite Oil

Apply this oil once a day to areas plagued by cellulite, and you'll start to see results quickly. Shake the jar gently before each use to recombine the oils.

Best for: Cellulite-prone areas

Tips: Pour the finished oil into a glass jar with a roll-on applicator top for ultimate convenience.

Store the finished oil away from light to keep its healing properties intact. This is a smart policy for all homemade oil mixtures.

Note: Exact measurements are important when you're making skin- and hair-care products. Turn to page 17 for how-tos.

3.5 oz	macadamia oil	100 g
1.8 oz	hazelnut oil	50 g
40	drops lemon essential oil	40
40	drops juniper essential oil	40
40	drops cypress essential oil	40
40	drops fennel essential oil	40
40	drops peppermint essential oil	40
40	drops cedar essential oil	40
40	drops grapefruit essential oil	40
40	drops patchouli essential oil	40

1. Pour macadamia oil, hazelnut oil, and lemon, juniper, cypress, fennel, peppermint, cedar, grapefruit and patchouli essential oils into a small glass bottle. Seal tightly.

2. Shake to combine.

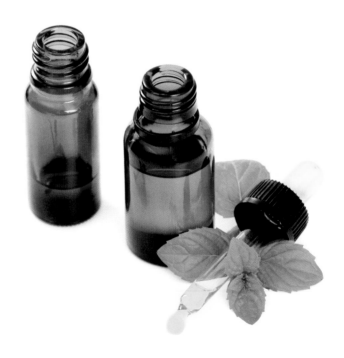

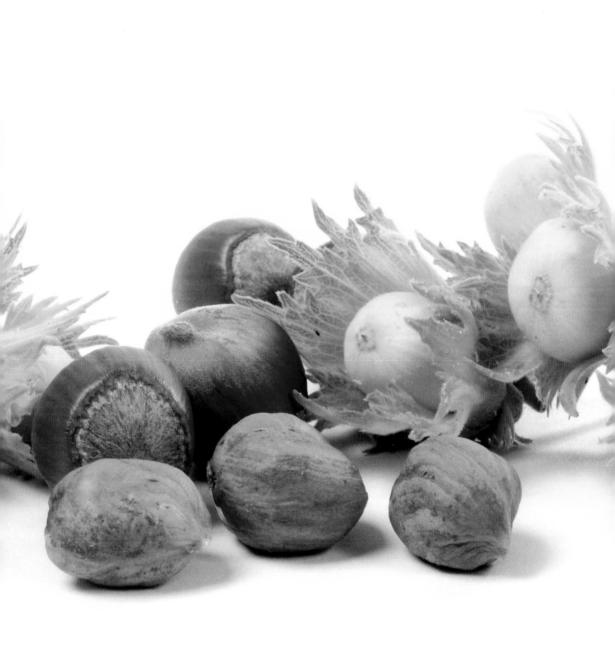

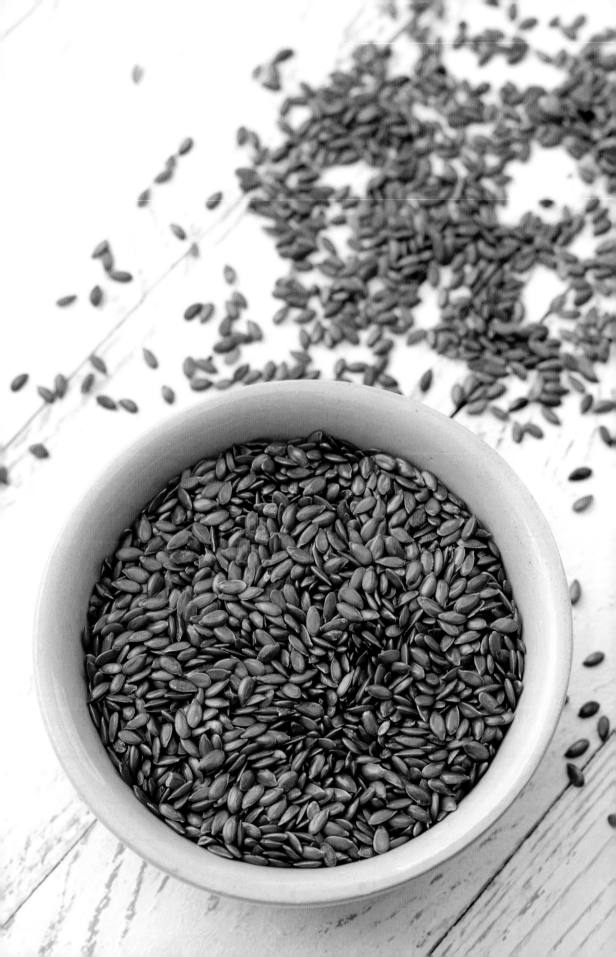

Flaxseed Oil

Flaxseed oil is soothing and makes skin beautiful — especially if you take it internally, as well. It's excellent for dry, sensitive and atopic skin.

Flaxseed oil (also called linseed oil in some parts of the world) is obtained from the seeds of the common flax plant *(Linum usitatissimum)*. It is an excellent source of essential fatty acids, especially polyunsaturated fatty acids — it contains about 58% alpha-linolenic acid (a type of omega-3 fatty acid) and about 15% linoleic acid (a type of omega-6 fatty acid). It also contains about 19% oleic acid (a type of monounsaturated fatty acid), the same type of good fat that olive oil offers. A 3.5-oz (100 g) portion of flaxseed oil also contains 17 mg of vitamin E, which is 113% of the recommended dietary allowance (RDA).

Used externally, flaxseed oil significantly improves dandruff, psoriasis, eczema and flaking skin. It is one of the most suitable oils for treating dry, sensitive and atopic (hypersensitive or allergy-prone) skin. This makes it ideal for use in cosmetics and for improving overall skin condition.

Flaxseed oil offers many benefits to the body when taken internally, and can help keep your skin looking and feeling good from the inside. (Although the focus here is on the oil's cosmetic properties, it doesn't hurt to remember that outer beauty begins with good nutrition.) In fact, for best results in acne treatment, flaxseed oil should be used both internally and externally. Nails, hair and scalp all benefit from the health-enhancing properties of this oil.

Flaxseed and Rose Moisturizing Face Cream

This concentrated cream is perfect for skin that requires extra hydration.

Best for: Dry to very dry skin

Tips: Rose water is often used in Middle Eastern and Mediterranean cooking. Look for it in Middle Eastern grocery stores and some well-stocked supermarkets.

You'll find pure vitamin E in liquid form at cosmetic-supply stores. It's also easy to buy online.

Note: Exact measurements are important when you're making skin- and hair-care products. Turn to page 17 for how-tos.

1.4 oz	flaxseed oil	40 g
0.2 oz	Lanette wax (see box, page 15)	6 g
0.1 oz	shea butter	3 g
0.07 oz	beeswax	2 g
5.1 oz	rose water (see tips, at left)	145 g
2	pinches citric acid powder (see box, page 27)	2
2	pinches ascorbic acid powder	2
0.18 oz	sweet almond oil	5 g
0.04 oz	pure vitamin E (see tips, at left)	1 g
10	drops grapefruit seed essential oil	10

1. Combine flaxseed oil, Lanette wax, shea butter and beeswax in a saucepan. Heat over low heat just until ingredients are completely melted. Remove from heat and keep warm.

2. Pour rose water into a separate saucepan. Heat until lukewarm. Using a wooden spoon, stir in citric acid and ascorbic acid until dissolved.

3. Stir rose water mixture into oil mixture. Using a hand mixer, beat at low speed for 1 to 2 minutes. Let stand for 10 minutes.

4. Stir in sweet almond oil, vitamin E and grapefruit seed essential oil. Using a hand mixer, beat at high speed for 1 minute.

5. Pour or spoon mixture into glass jars. Let cool.

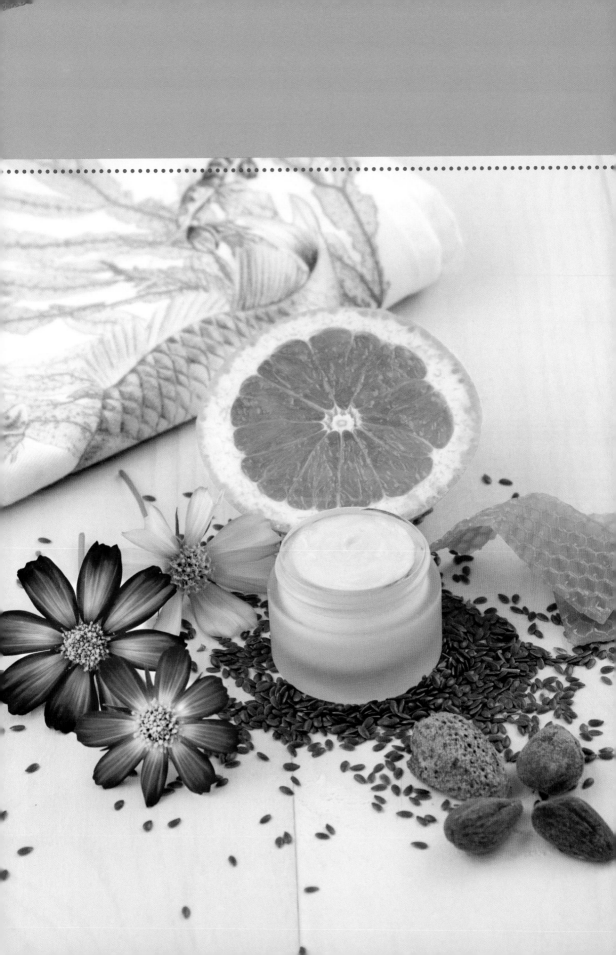

Flaxseed and Rose Hip Nourishing Face Cream

It is very important to nourish dry skin with creams like this. Apply it a few hours before going to bed so that it is well absorbed by the time your head hits the pillow.

Best for: Dry to extremely dry skin

Tip: Look for 100% pure beeswax that has been minimally processed. It is often sold in bulk, in chunks; if the recipe calls for a large amount, grate the wax so it will melt quickly and smoothly. Alternatively, you can buy beeswax that has been formed into pearls, which are easy to measure and melt quickly.

Note: Exact measurements are important when you're making skin- and hair-care products. Turn to page 17 for how-tos.

1.4 oz	flaxseed oil	40 g
0.2 oz	Lanette wax (see box, page 15)	6 g
0.1 oz	cocoa butter	3 g
0.07 oz	beeswax (see tip, at left)	2 g
0.07 oz	lanolin (see tip, page 76)	2 g
4.9 oz	orange flower water	140 g
2	pinches citric acid powder (see box, page 27)	2
2	pinches ascorbic acid powder	2
0.18 oz	rose hip seed oil	5 g
0.07 oz	pure vitamin A (see tip, opposite)	2 g
10	drops geranium essential oil	10

1. Combine flaxseed oil, Lanette wax, cocoa butter, beeswax and lanolin in a saucepan. Heat over low heat just until ingredients are completely melted. Remove from heat and keep warm.

2. Pour orange flower water into a separate saucepan. Heat until lukewarm. Using a wooden spoon, stir in citric acid and ascorbic acid until dissolved.

3. Stir orange flower water mixture into oil mixture. Using a hand mixer, beat at low speed for 1 to 2 minutes. Let stand for 10 minutes.

4. Stir in rose hip seed oil, vitamin A and geranium essential oil. Using a hand mixer, beat at high speed for 1 minute.

5. Pour or spoon mixture into glass jars. Let cool.

Flaxseed Extra-Sensitive Body Cream

Regular use of this gentle cream will bring considerable improvement to ultra-sensitive skin. It is excellent for soothing allergic reactions on the skin, too.

Best for: Atopic (hypersensitive or allergy-prone) skin

Tip: Liquid glycerin is a moisturizing ingredient often included in cosmetics, soaps, shampoos and creams. You'll find small bottles of it at drugstores, but cosmetic-supply stores sell larger bulk amounts.

Note: Exact measurements are important when you're making skin- and hair-care products. Turn to page 17 for how-tos.

1.8 oz	flaxseed oil	50 g
0.4 oz	Lanette wax (see box, page 15)	12 g
0.35 oz	castor oil	10 g
0.25 oz	shea butter	7 g
0.18 oz	beeswax (see tip, opposite)	5 g
0.1 oz	lanolin (see tip, page 76)	3 g
10.6 oz	rose water	300 g
4	pinches citric acid powder (see box, page 27)	4
4	pinches ascorbic acid powder	4
0.35 oz	liquid glycerin (see tip, at left)	10 g
0.07 oz	pure vitamin A (see tip, below)	2 g
0.07 oz	pure vitamin E	2 g
10	drops geranium essential oil	10

1. Combine flaxseed oil, Lanette wax, castor oil, shea butter, beeswax and lanolin in a saucepan. Heat over low heat just until ingredients are completely melted. Remove from heat and keep warm.

2. Pour rose water into a separate saucepan. Heat until lukewarm. Using a wooden spoon, stir in citric acid and ascorbic acid until dissolved.

3. Stir rose water mixture into oil mixture. Using a hand mixer, beat at low speed for 1 to 2 minutes. Let stand for 10 minutes.

4. Stir in glycerin, vitamins A and E, and geranium essential oil. Using a hand mixer, beat at high speed for 1 minute.

5. Pour or spoon mixture into glass jars. Let cool.

Tip: You'll find pure vitamins A and E in liquid form at cosmetic-supply stores. They are also easy to buy online.

Flaxseed and Collagen Body Cream

Skin can become parched if you don't care for it consistently. Use this cream after every shower to banish dryness.

Best for: Dry to very dry skin

Tip: Soluble collagen is a moisturizing ingredient that is often added to cosmetics. It comes in powder form at cosmetic-supply stores.

Note: Exact measurements are important when you're making skin- and hair-care products. Turn to page 17 for how-tos.

1.8 oz	flaxseed oil	50 g
0.4 oz	Lanette wax (see box, page 15)	12 g
0.35 oz	cocoa butter	10 g
0.18 oz	beeswax	5 g
0.18 oz	avocado oil (see tip, page 32)	5 g
0.07 oz	lanolin (see tip, below)	2 g
10.4 oz	mineral water	295 g
4	pinches citric acid powder (see box, page 27)	4
4	pinches ascorbic acid powder	4
0.35 oz	liquid glycerin	10 g
0.35 oz	soluble collagen (see tip, at left)	10 g
15	drops cedar essential oil	15

1. Combine flaxseed oil, Lanette wax, cocoa butter, beeswax, avocado oil and lanolin in a saucepan. Heat over low heat just until ingredients are completely melted. Remove from heat and keep warm.

2. Pour mineral water into a separate saucepan. Heat until lukewarm. Using a wooden spoon, stir in citric acid and ascorbic acid until dissolved.

3. Stir mineral water mixture into oil mixture. Using a hand mixer, beat at low speed for 1 to 2 minutes. Let stand for 10 minutes.

4. Stir in glycerin, collagen and cedar essential oil. Using a hand mixer, beat at high speed for 1 minute.

5. Pour or spoon mixture into glass jars. Let cool.

Tip: Lanolin is a waxy natural moisturizer derived from sheep's wool. It has long been used as a softening and moisturizing agent, especially in hand creams. You can find jars of it at cosmetic-supply stores. It has a distinctive, earthy aroma, and a little goes a long way.

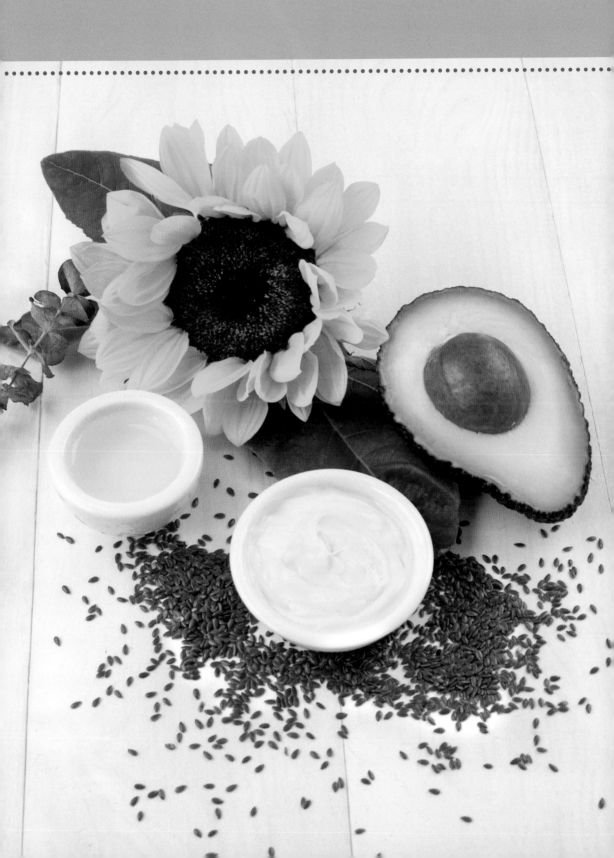

Flaxseed and Tea Tree Oil Nourishing Face Cream

Combining flaxseed, jojoba and coconut oils with tea tree essential oil creates the perfect acne-fighting moisturizer.

Best for: Acne-prone skin

Tip: Palmarosa essential oil may be a little less familiar than some essential oils, but its antibacterial properties make it a great tool for fighting acne. It also has a delicate floral scent that's similar to those of roses and geraniums.

Note: Exact measurements are important when you're making skin- and hair-care products. Turn to page 17 for how-tos.

Caution: Do not use rosemary essential oil if you have epilepsy or high blood pressure.

0.35 oz	flaxseed oil	10 g
0.2 oz	Lanette wax (see box, page 15)	6 g
0.18 oz	jojoba oil	5 g
0.1 oz	coconut oil	3 g
6 oz	mineral water	170 g
2	pinches citric acid powder (see box, page 27)	2
2	pinches ascorbic acid powder	2
10	drops tea tree essential oil	10
3	drops rosemary essential oil (see caution, at left)	3
3	drops palmarosa essential oil (see tip, at left)	3

1. Combine flaxseed oil, Lanette wax, jojoba oil and coconut oil in a saucepan. Heat over low heat just until ingredients are completely melted. Remove from heat and keep warm.

2. Pour mineral water into a separate saucepan. Heat until lukewarm. Using a wooden spoon, stir in citric acid and ascorbic acid until dissolved.

3. Stir mineral water mixture into oil mixture. Using a hand mixer, beat at low speed for 1 to 2 minutes. Let stand for 10 minutes.

4. Stir in tea tree, rosemary and palmarosa essential oils. Using a hand mixer, beat at high speed for 1 minute.

5. Pour or spoon mixture into glass jars. Let cool.

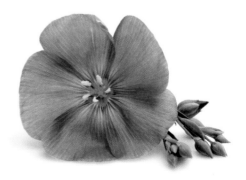

Flaxseed Moisturizing Hand Cream

This luxurious, rich cream pampers hands that are dry and chapped from manual labor. Slather on a generous amount and slip on cotton gloves for a softening overnight treatment.

Best for: Dry to very dry skin

Tip: Liquid glycerin is a moisturizing ingredient often included in cosmetics, soaps, shampoos and creams. You'll find small bottles of it at drugstores, but cosmetic-supply stores sell larger bulk amounts.

Note: Exact measurements are important when you're making skin- and hair-care products. Turn to page 17 for how-tos.

0.35 oz	flaxseed oil	10 g
0.25 oz	lanolin	7 g
0.2 oz	Lanette wax (see box, page 15)	6 g
0.18 oz	cocoa butter	5 g
0.18 oz	beeswax	5 g
5.8 oz	rose water	165 g
2	pinches citric acid powder (see box, page 27)	2
2	pinches ascorbic acid powder	2
0.18 oz	liquid glycerin (see tip, at left)	5 g
15	drops bay laurel essential oil (see tip, below)	15

1. Combine flaxseed oil, lanolin, Lanette wax, cocoa butter and beeswax in a saucepan. Heat over low heat just until ingredients are completely melted. Remove from heat and keep warm.

2. Pour rose water into a separate saucepan. Heat until lukewarm. Using a wooden spoon, stir in citric acid and ascorbic acid until dissolved.

3. Stir rose water mixture into oil mixture. Using a hand mixer, beat at low speed for 1 to 2 minutes. Let stand for 10 minutes.

4. Stir in glycerin and bay laurel essential oil. Using a hand mixer, beat at high speed for 1 minute.

5. Pour or spoon mixture into glass jars. Let cool.

Tip: Bay laurel is the name of the tree that produces the familiar bay leaves used in cooking. The essential oil distilled from the leaves has a spicy, very appealing scent.

Flaxseed and Chamomile Shower Gel

People are accustomed to strong but artificial scents. In contrast, the aroma of this homemade shower gel is subtle — and its fragrance is the least of its virtues. It cleanses and moisturizes at the same time, improving problem skin quickly.

Best for: Very dry or atopic (hypersensitive or allergy-prone) skin

Note: Exact measurements are important when you're making skin- and hair-care products. Turn to page 17 for how-tos.

10.6 oz	water	300 g
1.8 oz	glycerin soap base, chopped (see tips, below)	50 g
0.7 oz	flaxseed oil	20 g
0.35 oz	castor oil	10 g
20	drops chamomile essential oil	20

1. Pour water into a saucepan. Stir in glycerin soap base. Heat over low heat until soap base is dissolved. Remove from heat and let cool.

2. Stir in flaxseed oil, castor oil and chamomile essential oil. Pour into a bottle (see tips, below).

Tips: Glycerin soap base is often labeled "melt and pour" in stores that sell soap-making supplies, because crafters use it as the foundation for homemade soaps that are melted and poured into molds. It comes in large bars that range in size from 1 lb to 3½ lbs (500 g to 1.75 kg). Cut off a chunk and chop just the amount you need for the recipe.

Pour the finished shower gel into a pump dispenser for ultimate convenience.

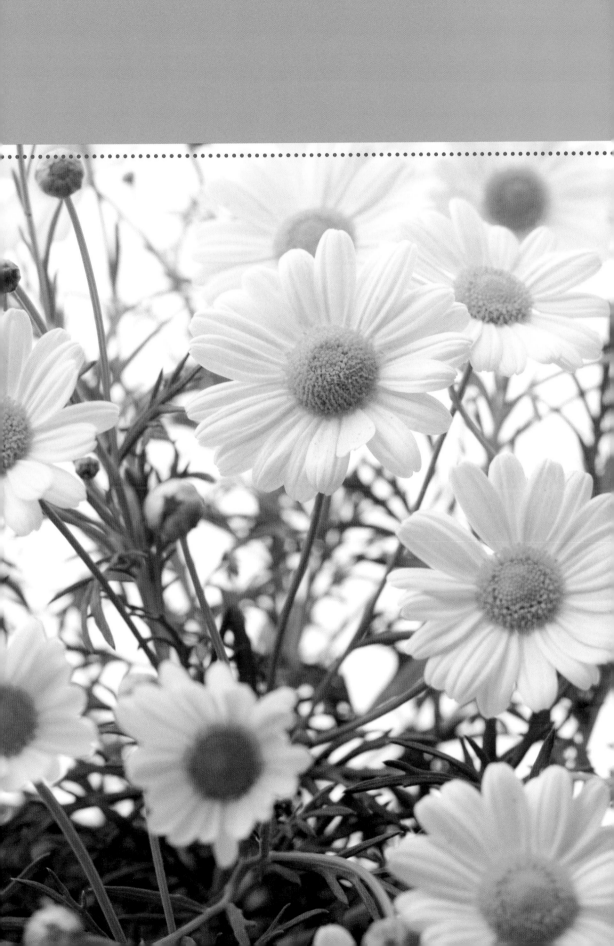

Flaxseed Face and Body Oil

As with any oil mixture, make sure to give the bottle a gentle shake before use to ensure this mixture is uniformly blended. Apply once or twice a day to the affected area for soothing relief.

Best for: Psoriasis, eczema and flaky skin

3.5 oz	flaxseed oil	100 g
1.8 oz	St. John's wort oil	50 g
15	drops myrrh essential oil	15
15	drops chamomile essential oil (see tip, below)	15

1. Pour flaxseed oil, St. John's wort oil, and myrrh and chamomile essential oils into a small glass bottle. Seal tightly.

2. Shake to combine.

Tip: You'll often find two types of chamomile essential oil at cosmetic-supply stores: German and Roman. They come from different strains of the chamomile plant, but both are soothing additions to homemade skin- and hair-care products.

Flaxseed and Wheat Germ Flaky Scalp Oil

Moisten a cotton swab with water, then use it to rub this oil over the area you want to treat. Apply it at night and wash your hair as usual in the morning.

Best for: Dandruff-prone or dry, flaky scalps

0.7 oz	flaxseed oil	20 g
0.18 oz	rosemary essential oil (see caution, opposite)	5 g
0.15 oz	wheat germ oil (see tip, page 96)	4 g
0.1 oz	marjoram essential oil	3 g

1. Pour flaxseed oil, rosemary essential oil, wheat germ oil and marjoram essential oil into a small glass bottle. Seal tightly.

2. Shake to combine.

Flaxseed and Rosemary Dandruff Shampoo

Use this fresh-smelling natural shampoo to chase away flakes and banish dryness. Shake gently before each use to mix the oils well.

Best for:
Dandruff-prone or dry, flaky scalps

Tip: Coco betaine (short for cocamido-propyl betaine) is a surfactant made from coconut oil and gives shampoos their cleaning power and lather. It's easy to find at cosmetic-supply stores.

Note: Exact measurements are important when you're making skin- and hair-care products. Turn to page 17 for how-tos.

Caution: Do not use rosemary essential oil if you have epilepsy or high blood pressure.

2 tbsp	fresh or dried rosemary	30 mL
7.2 oz	mineral water	205 g
5.3 oz	coco betaine (see tip, at left)	150 g
0.35 oz	flaxseed oil	10 g
0.35 oz	cider vinegar	10 g
25	drops rosemary essential oil (see caution, at left)	25
10	drops sage essential oil	10
10	drops lemon essential oil	10

1. Place rosemary in a heatproof bowl. In a saucepan, bring mineral water to a boil. Pour boiling mineral water over rosemary. Cover and let steep for 10 minutes.

2. Using a fine-mesh sieve lined with cheesecloth, strain the infusion into a clean bowl. Let cool completely.

3. Pour rosemary infusion, coco betaine, flaxseed oil, cider vinegar, and rosemary, sage and lemon essential oils into a bottle. Seal tightly.

4. Shake gently to combine.

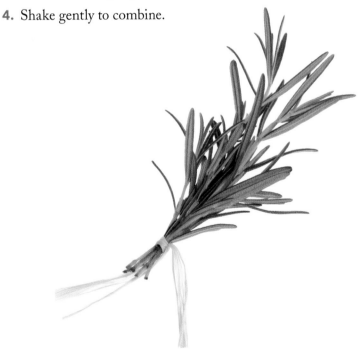

Flaxseed Cracked-Skin Ointment

This cream is designed to treat painful skin cracks that plague the elbows, knees and heels. Apply it daily for a few days, then once or twice a week or as often as necessary to keep the skin soft and supple.

Best for: Cracked skin, especially at the elbows, knees and heels

Tip: Look for 100% pure beeswax that has been minimally processed. It is often sold in bulk, in chunks; if the recipe calls for a large amount, grate the wax so it will melt quickly and smoothly. Alternatively, you can buy beeswax that has been formed into pearls, which are easy to measure and melt quickly.

Note: Exact measurements are important when you're making skin- and hair-care products. Turn to page 17 for how-tos.

0.35 oz	flaxseed oil	10 g
0.35 oz	beeswax (see tip, at left)	10 g
0.2 oz	Lanette wax (see box, page 15)	6 g
1.4 oz	lanolin	40 g
4 oz	mineral water	115 g
2	pinches citric acid powder (see box, page 27)	2
2	pinches ascorbic acid powder	2
0.7 oz	liquid glycerin	20 g
20	drops tea tree essential oil (see tip, below)	20

1. Combine flaxseed oil, beeswax, Lanette wax and lanolin in a saucepan. Heat over low heat just until ingredients are completely melted. Remove from heat and keep warm.

2. Pour mineral water into a separate saucepan. Heat until lukewarm. Using a wooden spoon, stir in citric acid and ascorbic acid until dissolved.

3. Stir mineral water mixture into oil mixture. Using a hand mixer, beat at low speed for 1 to 2 minutes. Let stand for 10 minutes.

4. Stir in glycerin and tea tree essential oil. Using a hand mixer, beat at high speed for 1 minute.

5. Pour or spoon mixture into glass jars. Let cool.

Tip: The essential oils you use for skin- and hair-care products must be 100% pure. Don't use synthetic scents or oils, or essences used in fragrance burners or lamp rings.

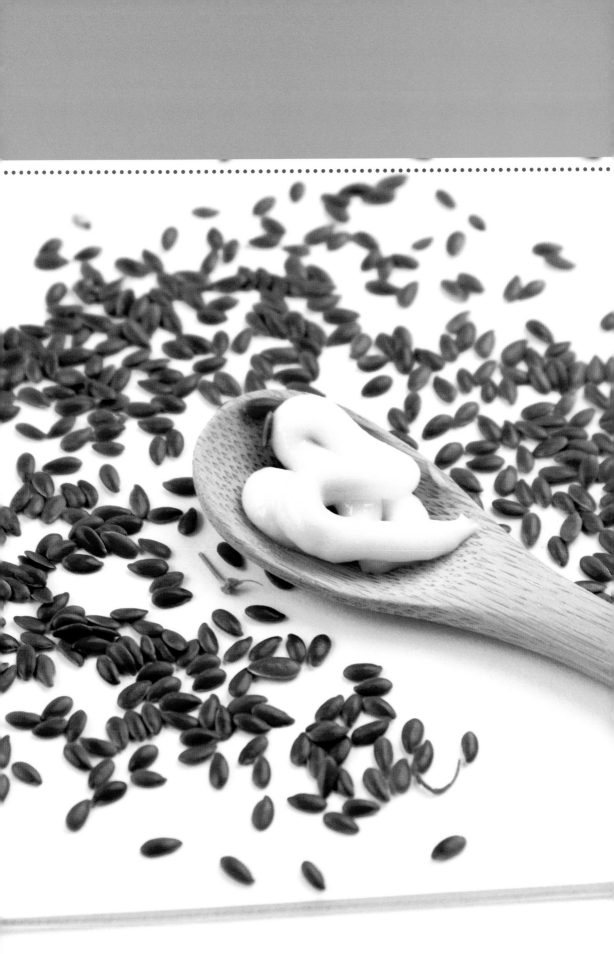

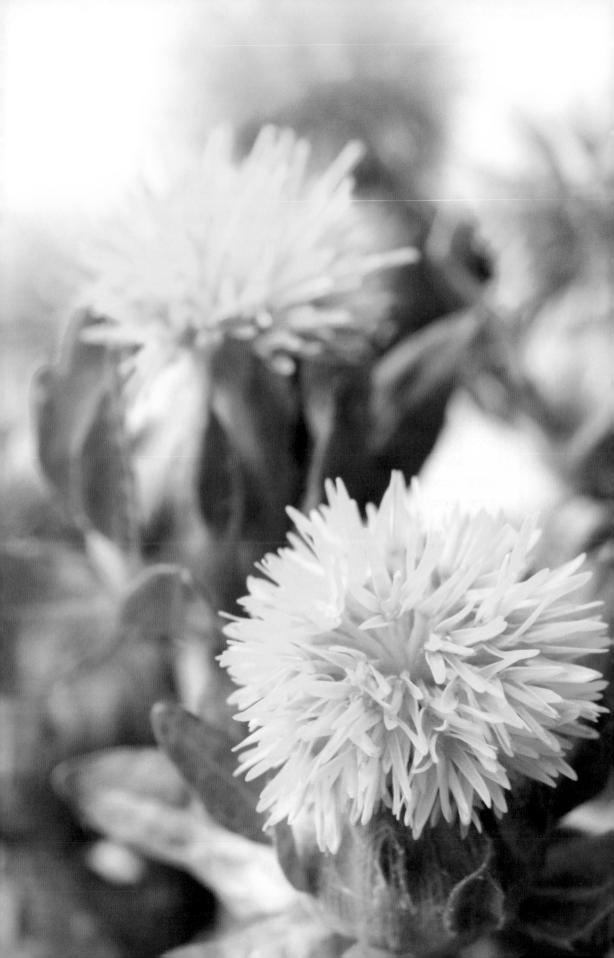

Safflower Oil

Safflower oil helps prevent and heal split ends, which are caused by dryness at the tip of the hair shaft. Using it is an easy fix for a common problem for people with dry, fragile hair.

Safflower oil is obtained from the seeds of the thistle *Carthamus tinctorius,* which is native to India. This oil is prized in Asian cuisine and is used widely in cooking.

There are two types of safflower oil, which differ in the proportions of polyunsaturated and monounsaturated fatty acids they contain. For the recipes in this book, use the type that contains more polyunsaturates: it should contain about 75% polyunsaturated fatty acids (omega-6 linoleic acid) and 15% monounsaturated fatty acids (omega-9 oleic acid).

This oil is rich in vitamin E (alpha-tocopherol). A 3.5-oz (100 g) portion contains 34 mg of vitamin E, or more than 250% of the recommended dietary allowance (RDA). It has a considerable phytosterol content, as well (442 mg per 3.5-oz/100 g portion). These plant-based sterols help regulate blood cholesterol levels.

Safflower oil is excellent for firming and toning the skin, actively assists in the removal of fat deposits (cellulite) and combats dermatitis all over the body. When it is gently warmed, the oil is ideal for moisturizing the cuticles, which are the foundation of beautiful nails. If your cuticles are dry, ripped or excessively thickened, the nails will grow unevenly and will often develop ridges that need to be polished down.

Safflower Fluid Retention Treatment Cream

The most common areas troubled by fluid retention are the legs and the belly. Massage this cream gently into the skin over the areas you want to treat.

Best for: Swollen or cellulite-prone areas

Tip: Store essential oils in a cool, dark place. Light exposure can diminish their healing properties.

Note: Exact measurements are important when you're making skin- and hair-care products. Turn to page 17 for how-tos.

1 oz	safflower oil	30 g
0.4 oz	Lanette wax (see box, page 15)	12 g
0.18 oz	cocoa butter	5 g
12.3 oz	mineral water	350 g
4	pinches citric acid powder (see box, page 27)	4
4	pinches ascorbic acid powder	4
15	drops fennel essential oil (see tip, at left)	15
15	drops geranium essential oil	15
15	drops grapefruit essential oil	15
10	drops eucalyptus essential oil	10

1. Combine safflower oil, Lanette wax and cocoa butter in a saucepan. Heat over low heat just until ingredients are completely melted. Remove from heat and keep warm.

2. Pour mineral water into a separate saucepan. Heat until lukewarm. Using a wooden spoon, stir in citric acid and ascorbic acid until dissolved.

3. Stir mineral water mixture into oil mixture. Using a hand mixer, beat at low speed for 1 to 2 minutes. Let stand for 10 minutes.

4. Stir in fennel, geranium, grapefruit and eucalyptus essential oils. Using a hand mixer, beat at high speed for 1 minute.

5. Pour or spoon mixture into glass jars. Let cool.

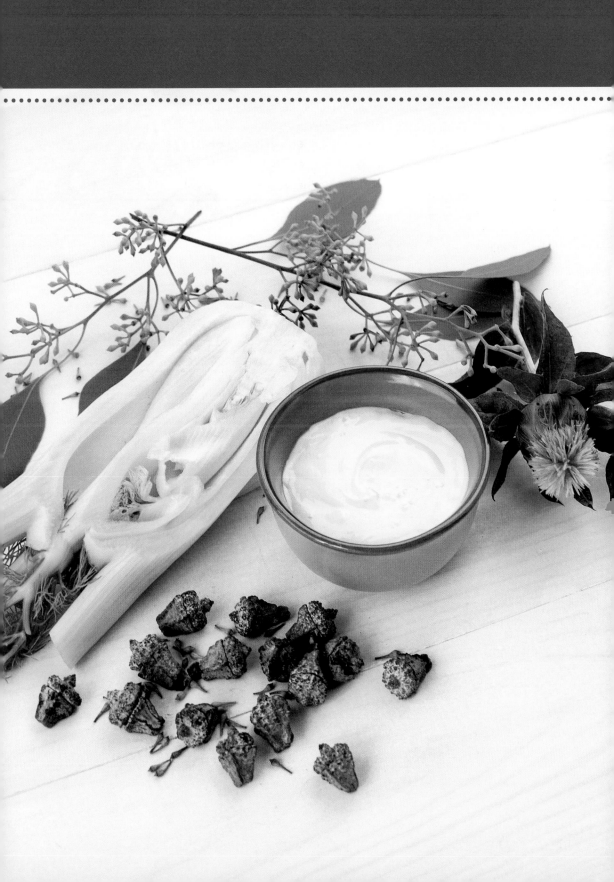

Safflower Cellulite-Fighting Cream

Apply this silky cream to areas where fat accumulates. It improves the appearance of cellulite or jiggly areas that require a bit of firming.

Best for: Fatty or cellulite-prone areas

Tip: Look for chunks or blocks of pure cocoa butter at cosmetic-supply stores. If you're using a large amount in a recipe, chop it up before adding it to the saucepan so it will melt more quickly.

Note: Exact measurements are important when you're making skin- and hair-care products. Turn to page 17 for how-tos.

Caution: Do not use rosemary essential oil if you have epilepsy or high blood pressure.

1 oz	safflower oil	30 g
0.4 oz	Lanette wax (see box, page 15)	12 g
0.18 oz	cocoa butter (see tip, at left)	5 g
12.3 oz	mineral water	350 g
4	pinches citric acid powder (see box, page 27)	4
4	pinches ascorbic acid powder	4
10	drops rosemary essential oil (see caution, at left)	10
10	drops juniper essential oil (see tip, below)	10
10	drops ginger essential oil	10
10	drops lemon essential oil	10
10	drops cypress essential oil	10
10	drops geranium essential oil	10

1. Combine safflower oil, Lanette wax and cocoa butter in a saucepan. Heat over low heat just until ingredients are completely melted. Remove from heat and keep warm.

2. Pour mineral water into a separate saucepan. Heat until lukewarm. Using a wooden spoon, stir in citric acid and ascorbic acid until dissolved.

3. Stir mineral water mixture into oil mixture. Using a hand mixer, beat at low speed for 1 to 2 minutes. Let stand for 10 minutes.

4. Stir in rosemary, juniper, ginger, lemon, cypress and geranium essential oils. Using a hand mixer, beat at high speed for 1 minute.

5. Pour or spoon mixture into glass jars. Let cool.

Tip: The essential oils you use for skin- and hair-care products must be 100% pure. Don't use synthetic scents or oils, or essences designed for use in fragrance burners or lamp rings.

Safflower and Tea Tree Cuticle Cream

Apply a small amount of this refreshing cream to damaged cuticles every night before you go to bed, massaging it in circles. Once they're healed, your cuticles will need this treatment only once a week for maintenance.

Best for: Dry and/or ragged cuticles

Tip: When your cuticles are in good shape, they'll need to be pushed back off the nails from time to time as they grow. Gently push them with the sloped end of an orange stick, a special wooden tool created for this purpose (the pointed end is for cleaning under the nails). You can buy orange sticks in drugstores and online.

0.7 oz	safflower oil	20 g
0.2 oz	Lanette wax (see box, page 15)	6 g
0.18 oz	shea butter (see tip, below)	5 g
0.18 oz	lanolin	5 g
0.1 oz	beeswax	3 g
5.6 oz	mineral water	160 g
2	pinches citric acid powder (see box, page 27)	2
2	pinches ascorbic acid powder	2
10	drops tea tree essential oil	10

1. Combine safflower oil, Lanette wax, shea butter, lanolin and beeswax in a saucepan. Heat over low heat just until ingredients are completely melted. Remove from heat and keep warm.

2. Pour mineral water into a separate saucepan. Heat until lukewarm. Using a wooden spoon, stir in citric acid and ascorbic acid until dissolved.

3. Stir mineral water mixture into oil mixture. Using a hand mixer, beat at low speed for 1 to 2 minutes. Let stand for 10 minutes.

4. Stir in tea tree essential oil. Using a hand mixer, beat at high speed for 1 minute.

5. Pour or spoon mixture into glass jars. Let cool.

Tip: Pure shea butter comes in chunks, like cocoa butter, at cosmetic-supply stores. Break or chop it up before adding it to the saucepan so that it melts quickly and easily.

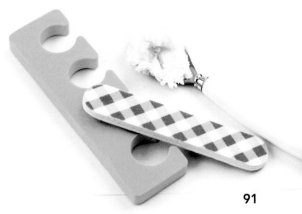

Safflower Dermatitis-Fighting Cream

Dermatitis is a common condition characterized by swollen, sore and reddened skin. For relief, apply this soothing cream to the affected area once a day. You'll quickly see (and feel) improvement.

Best for: Red, irritated skin

Tip: Look for 100% pure beeswax that has been minimally processed. It is often sold in bulk, in chunks; if the recipe calls for a large amount, grate the wax so it will melt quickly and smoothly. Alternatively, you can buy beeswax that has been formed into pearls, which are easy to measure and melt quickly.

Note: Exact measurements are important when you're making skin- and hair-care products. Turn to page 17 for how-tos.

0.5 oz	safflower oil	15 g
0.2 oz	Lanette wax (see box, page 15)	6 g
0.18 oz	cocoa butter	5 g
0.18 oz	lanolin (see tip, below)	5 g
0.07 oz	beeswax (see tip, at left)	2 g
5.8 oz	witch hazel	165 g
2	pinches citric acid powder (see box, page 27)	2
2	pinches ascorbic acid powder	2
15	drops cedar essential oil	15
5	drops tea tree essential oil	5
5	drops bergamot essential oil	5

1. Combine safflower oil, Lanette wax, cocoa butter, lanolin and beeswax in a saucepan. Heat over low heat just until ingredients are completely melted. Remove from heat and keep warm.

2. Pour witch hazel into a separate saucepan. Heat until lukewarm. Using a wooden spoon, stir in citric acid and ascorbic acid until dissolved.

3. Stir witch hazel mixture into oil mixture. Using a hand mixer, beat at low speed for 1 to 2 minutes. Let stand for 10 minutes.

4. Stir in cedar, tea tree and bergamot essential oils. Using a hand mixer, beat at high speed for 1 minute.

5. Pour or spoon mixture into glass jars. Let cool.

Tip: Lanolin is a waxy natural moisturizer derived from sheep's wool. It has long been used as a softening and moisturizing agent, especially in hand creams. You can find jars of it at cosmetic-supply stores. It has a distinctive, earthy aroma, and a little goes a long way.

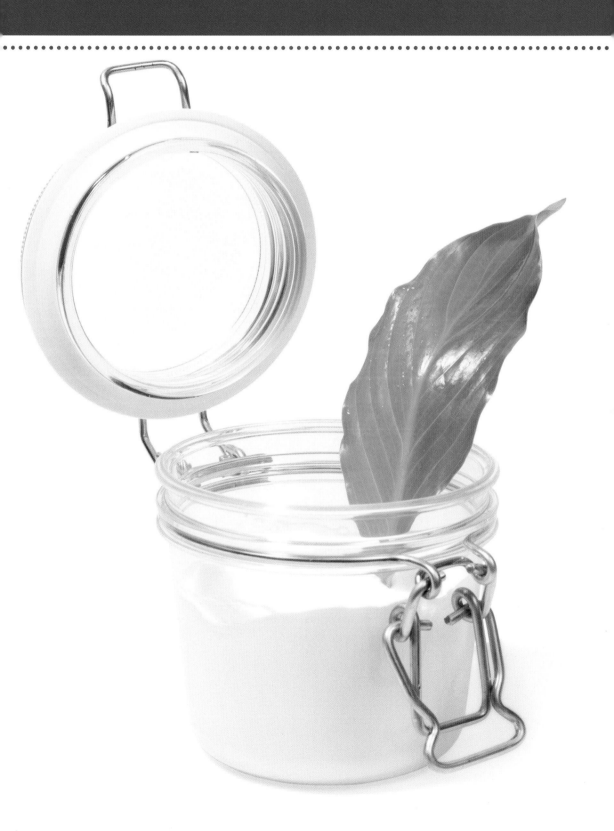

Safflower and Patchouli Firming Face Cream

This is the ideal firming cream for all skin types. It's gentle and very agreeable, so it's especially good for people whose skin won't tolerate other cosmetics.

Best for: All skin types

Tips: Orange flower water is also called orange blossom water. You'll find it in Middle Eastern grocery stores and some well-stocked supermarkets, where it's sold for use in cooking.

Look for pure vitamin A in liquid form at cosmetic-supply stores. It's also easy to buy online.

Note: Exact measurements are important when you're making skin- and hair-care products. Turn to page 17 for how-tos.

0.7 oz	safflower oil	20 g
0.4 oz	sesame oil	12 g
0.2 oz	Lanette wax (see box, page 15)	6 g
0.18 oz	cocoa butter (see tips, opposite)	5 g
5.3 oz	orange flower water (see tips, at left)	150 g
2	pinches citric acid powder (see box, page 27)	2
2	pinches ascorbic acid powder	2
0.15 oz	pure vitamin A (see tips, at left)	4 g
10	drops patchouli essential oil	10

1. Combine safflower oil, sesame oil, Lanette wax and cocoa butter in a saucepan. Heat over low heat just until ingredients are completely melted. Remove from heat and keep warm.

2. Pour orange flower water into a separate saucepan. Heat until lukewarm. Using a wooden spoon, stir in citric acid and ascorbic acid until dissolved.

3. Stir orange flower water mixture into oil mixture. Using a hand mixer, beat at low speed for 1 to 2 minutes. Let stand for 10 minutes.

4. Stir in vitamin A and patchouli essential oil. Using a hand mixer, beat at high speed for 1 minute.

5. Pour or spoon mixture into glass jars. Let cool.

Safflower Firming Body Cream

This lemony, herb-scented cream absorbs readily into the skin, making it ideal to use just after a shower.

Best for: All skin types

Tips: Look for chunks or blocks of pure cocoa butter at cosmetic-supply stores. If you're using a large amount in a recipe, chop it up before adding it to the saucepan so it will melt more quickly.

Liquid glycerin is a moisturizing ingredient often included in cosmetics, soaps, shampoos and creams. You'll find small bottles of it at drugstores, but cosmetic-supply stores sell larger bulk amounts.

Note: Exact measurements are important when you're making skin- and hair-care products. Turn to page 17 for how-tos.

0.7 oz	safflower oil	20 g
0.4 oz	Lanette wax (see box, page 15)	12 g
0.35 oz	cocoa butter (see tips, at left)	10 g
0.18 oz	hazelnut oil	5 g
0.18 oz	St. John's wort oil	5 g
11.8 oz	mineral water	335 g
4	pinches citric acid powder (see box, page 27)	4
4	pinches ascorbic acid powder	4
0.35 oz	liquid glycerin (see tips, at left)	10 g
20	drops lemongrass essential oil	20
20	drops frankincense essential oil	20

1. Combine safflower oil, Lanette wax, cocoa butter, hazelnut oil and St. John's wort oil in a saucepan. Heat over low heat just until ingredients are completely melted. Remove from heat and keep warm.

2. Pour mineral water into a separate saucepan. Heat until lukewarm. Using a wooden spoon, stir in citric acid and ascorbic acid until dissolved.

3. Stir mineral water mixture into oil mixture. Using a hand mixer, beat at low speed for 1 to 2 minutes. Let stand for 10 minutes.

4. Stir in glycerin, and lemongrass and frankincense essential oils. Using a hand mixer, beat at high speed for 1 minute.

5. Pour or spoon mixture into glass jars. Let cool.

Safflower and Wheat Germ Oil Eye Cream

This cream is highly recommended to reduce crow's-feet in mature skin, but it is also useful for younger skin suffering from premature dryness around the eyes.

Best for:
Mature skin

Tip: Wheat germ oil is highly perishable. Store it in the refrigerator to keep it from going rancid.

Note: Exact measurements are important when you're making skin- and hair-care products. Turn to page 17 for how-tos.

0.35 oz	safflower oil	10 g
0.35 oz	wheat germ oil (see tip, at left)	10 g
0.1 oz	Lanette wax (see box, page 15)	3 g
2.8 oz	orange flower water	80 g
1	pinch ascorbic acid powder (see box, page 27)	1
4	drops geranium essential oil	4

1. Combine safflower oil, wheat germ oil and Lanette wax in a saucepan. Heat over low heat just until ingredients are completely melted. Remove from heat and keep warm.

2. Pour orange flower water into a separate saucepan. Heat until lukewarm. Using a wooden spoon, stir in ascorbic acid until dissolved.

3. Stir orange flower water mixture into oil mixture. Using a hand mixer, beat at low speed for 1 to 2 minutes. Let stand for 10 minutes.

4. Stir in geranium essential oil. Using a hand mixer, beat at high speed for 1 minute.

5. Pour or spoon mixture into glass jars. Let cool.

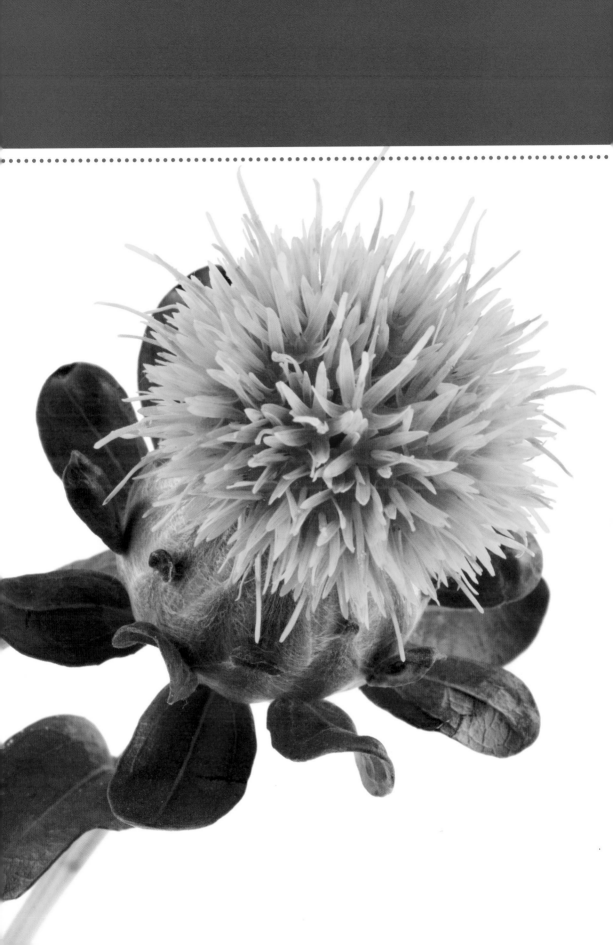

Safflower Oil Dermatitis Treatment

For quick relief, apply a small amount of this oil once a day to areas affected by dermatitis. It will relax the senses, too, with its fragrant blend of essential oils.

Best for: Red, irritated skin

Tip: Choose extra-virgin or virgin oils made from the first cold pressing.

Note: Exact measurements are important when you're making skin- and hair-care products. Turn to page 17 for how-tos.

1.8 oz	safflower oil	50 g
0.25 oz	olive oil (see tip, at left)	7 g
0.04 oz	marjoram essential oil	1 g
3	drops lavender essential oil	3
3	drops ginger essential oil	3

1. Pour safflower oil, olive oil, and marjoram, lavender and ginger essential oils into a small glass bottle. Seal tightly.
2. Shake to combine.

Safflower Oil for Damaged or Tired Hair

Pure safflower oil on its own is an excellent hair treatment. Apply a few drops to the ends of each section you want to treat, then massage the oil in with your fingertips. Wrap your hair in a towel and leave it on overnight. Wash your hair as usual in the morning.

Safflower Anti-Cellulite Body Oil

This heady, aromatic oil is the perfect solution for firming up dimpled areas on the abdomen and thighs. Combine it with an energizing massage for excellent results.

Best for: Cellulite-prone areas

Tips: The essential oils you use for skin- and hair-care products must be 100% pure. Don't use synthetic scents or oils, or essences used in fragrance burners or lamp rings.

Store the finished oil away from light to keep its healing properties intact. This is a smart policy for all homemade oils.

Note: Exact measurements are important when you're making skin- and hair-care products. Turn to page 17 for how-tos.

5.3 oz	safflower oil	150 g
30	drops geranium essential oil (see tips, at left)	30
30	drops grapefruit essential oil	30
30	drops cypress essential oil	30
30	drops fennel essential oil	30
30	drops peppermint essential oil	30
30	drops cedar essential oil	30
30	drops lemongrass essential oil	30

1. Pour safflower oil, and geranium, grapefruit, cypress, fennel, peppermint, cedar and lemongrass essential oils into a small glass bottle. Seal tightly.

2. Shake to combine.

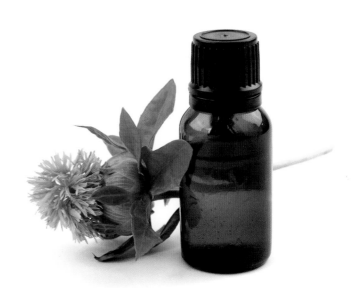

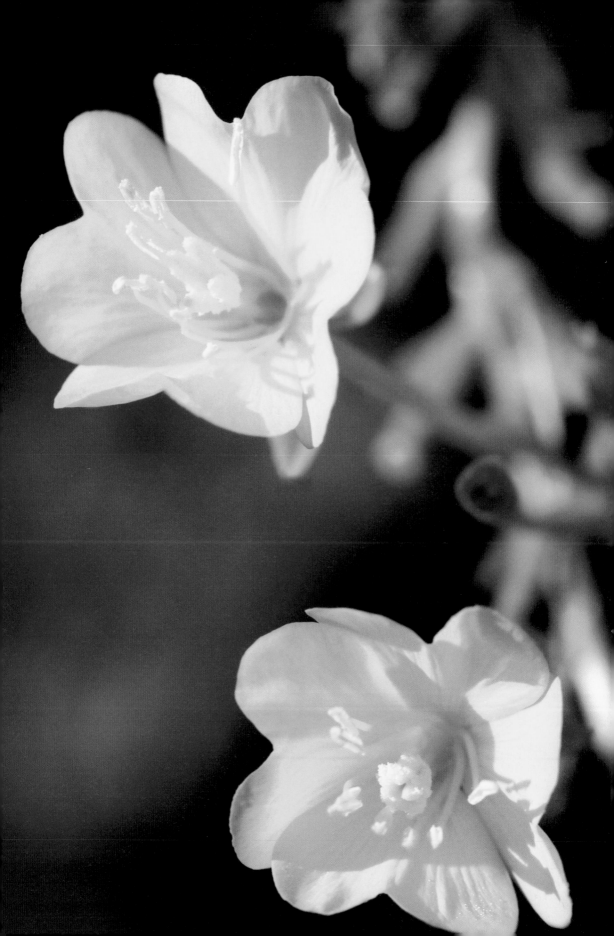

Evening Primrose Oil

Evening primrose oil is often used to treat acne, and can be applied topically or taken orally.

Evening primrose *(Oenothera biennis)* belongs to the family Onagraceae and is sometimes called evening star or sundrop. It is native to the Americas but was introduced to Europe in the 17th century. Native North Americans used the plant internally to treat asthma. They also used it externally to relieve skin problems and heal wounds. Today, the evening primrose plant is cultivated mainly for its oil, which is extracted from the seeds via cold pressing. The oil contains nearly all the active ingredients of the plant and a number of beneficial substances — most notably, fatty acids, including linoleic, gamma-linolenic, oleic, palmitic and stearic acids.

The cosmetic uses of evening primrose oil are many and varied, because it contains substances that help with contrasting problems. For example, one of the most outstanding qualities of this oil is its moisturizing ability, which makes it perfect for use on dry skin. But, at the same time, evening primrose oil can dilute oils that accumulate in the pores, which helps reduce acne. It also helps relieve the symptoms of eczema and noticeably improves muscle strains and tears.

Rubbed gently over the skin, evening primrose oil is a good tool in the treatment of Raynaud's disease, which causes circulatory problems in the toes, fingers, ears and nose. Massaging the affected areas with evening primrose oil helps improve circulation and prevents pain and reddening of the skin.

Evening primrose oil is sold in soft gel capsules at the pharmacy, in the vitamin aisle. You can also find vials or small bottles of the oil at some cosmetic-supply stores. No matter what form you choose, be sure to choose a trusted brand. To use the oil in these recipes, you'll have to pierce the capsules with a needle and squeeze out the contents. Generally, two 500 mg gel capsules will yield about 0.04 oz (1 g) evening primrose oil.

Evening Primrose Moisturizing Face Cream

Tight, parched skin will drink in this emollient cream and ask for more. Keep it close at hand in the cold weather, when skin is drier.

Best for: Dry skin

Tips: Use a large, sharp sewing needle to pierce the evening primrose oil capsules so you can squeeze out the contents. The bigger the hole, the faster the process will go.

Look for 100% pure beeswax that has been minimally processed. It is often sold in bulk, in chunks; if the recipe calls for a large amount, grate the wax so it will melt quickly and smoothly. Alternatively, you can buy beeswax that has been formed into pearls, which are easy to measure and melt quickly.

20	capsules (each 500 mg) evening primrose oil	20
0.35 oz	sweet almond oil	10 g
0.25 oz	cocoa butter	7 g
0.2 oz	Lanette wax (see box, page 15)	6 g
0.15 oz	beeswax (see tips, at left)	4 g
5.6 oz	rose water	160 g
2	pinches citric acid powder (see box, page 27)	2
2	pinches ascorbic acid powder	2
0.18 oz	liquid glycerin	5 g
5	drops grapefruit essential oil	5

1. Using a large needle, pierce evening primrose oil capsules and squeeze the contents into a saucepan (see tips, at left). Add sweet almond oil, cocoa butter, Lanette wax and beeswax. Heat over low heat just until ingredients are completely melted. Remove from heat and keep warm.

2. Pour rose water into a separate saucepan. Heat until lukewarm. Using a wooden spoon, stir in citric acid and ascorbic acid until dissolved.

3. Stir rose water mixture into oil mixture. Using a hand mixer, beat at low speed for 1 to 2 minutes. Let stand for 10 minutes.

4. Stir in glycerin and grapefruit essential oil. Using a hand mixer, beat at high speed for 1 minute.

5. Pour or spoon mixture into glass jars. Let cool.

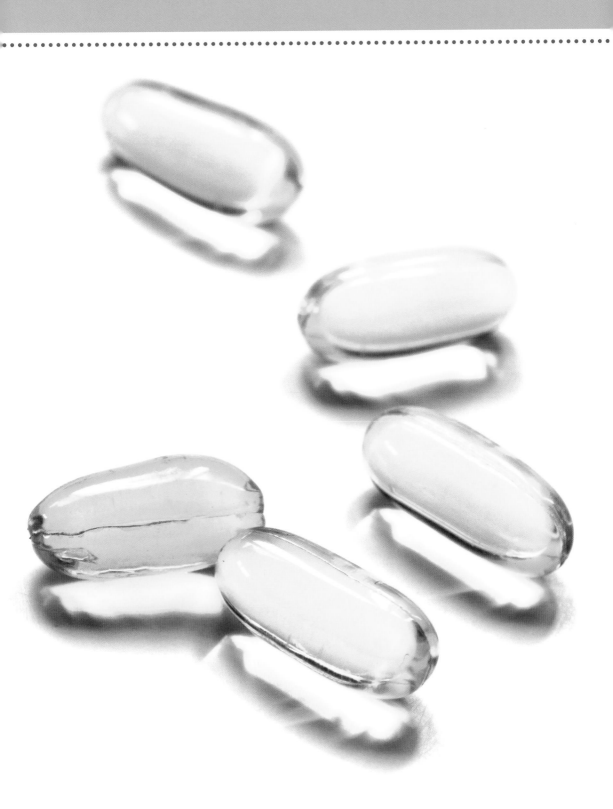

Evening Primrose Nourishing Face Cream

This is an ideal night cream. For best results, apply it two hours before retiring so it will be thoroughly absorbed before your face touches the pillow.

Best for: Dry skin

Tips: Use a large, sharp sewing needle to pierce the evening primrose oil capsules so you can squeeze out the contents. The bigger the hole, the faster the process will go.

Pure shea butter comes in chunks, like cocoa butter, at cosmetic-supply stores. Break or chop it up before adding it to the saucepan so that it melts quickly and easily.

Note: Exact measurements are important when you're making skin- and hair-care products. Turn to page 17 for how-tos.

25	capsules (each 500 mg) evening primrose oil	25
0.2 oz	Lanette wax (see box, page 15)	6 g
0.18 oz	avocado oil	5 g
0.18 oz	flaxseed oil	5 g
0.18 oz	shea butter (see tips, at left)	5 g
0.1 oz	beeswax	3 g
0.1 oz	lanolin	3 g
5.8 oz	mineral water	165 g
2	pinches citric acid powder (see box, page 27)	2
2	pinches ascorbic acid powder	2
10	drops chamomile essential oil (see tip, below)	10

1. Using a large needle, pierce evening primrose oil capsules and squeeze the contents into a saucepan (see tips, at left). Add Lanette wax, avocado oil, flaxseed oil, shea butter, beeswax and lanolin. Heat over low heat just until ingredients are completely melted. Remove from heat and keep warm.

2. Pour mineral water into a separate saucepan. Heat until lukewarm. Using a wooden spoon, stir in citric acid and ascorbic acid until dissolved.

3. Stir mineral water mixture into oil mixture. Using a hand mixer, beat at low speed for 1 to 2 minutes. Let stand for 10 minutes.

4. Stir in chamomile essential oil. Using a hand mixer, beat at high speed for 1 minute.

5. Pour or spoon mixture into glass jars. Let cool.

Tip: You'll often find two types of chamomile essential oil at cosmetic-supply stores: German and Roman. They come from different strains of the chamomile plant, but both are soothing additions to homemade skin- and hair-care products.

Evening Primrose Moisturizing Body Cream

If you have dry skin, the best way to treat and protect it is to diligently moisturize every day. This cream will help you enjoy the job.

Best for: Dry skin

Tip: Liquid glycerin is a moisturizing ingredient often included in cosmetics, soaps, shampoos and creams. You'll find small bottles of it at drugstores, but cosmetic-supply stores sell larger bulk amounts.

Note: Exact measurements are important when you're making skin- and hair-care products. Turn to page 17 for how-tos.

20	capsules (each 500 mg) evening primrose oil	20
0.4 oz	Lanette wax (see box, page 15)	12 g
0.35 oz	hazelnut oil	10 g
0.35 oz	sweet almond oil	10 g
0.35 oz	cocoa butter	10 g
11.8 oz	mineral water	335 g
4	pinches citric acid powder (see box, page 27)	4
4	pinches ascorbic acid powder	4
0.35 oz	liquid glycerin (see tip, at left)	10 g
15	drops lavender essential oil	15

1. Using a large needle, pierce evening primrose oil capsules and squeeze the contents into a saucepan (see tips, opposite). Add Lanette wax, hazelnut oil, sweet almond oil and cocoa butter. Heat over low heat just until ingredients are completely melted. Remove from heat and keep warm.

2. Pour mineral water into a separate saucepan. Heat until lukewarm. Using a wooden spoon, stir in citric acid and ascorbic acid until dissolved.

3. Stir mineral water mixture into oil mixture. Using a hand mixer, beat at low speed for 1 to 2 minutes. Let stand for 10 minutes.

4. Stir in glycerin and lavender essential oil. Using a hand mixer, beat at high speed for 1 minute.

5. Pour or spoon mixture into glass jars. Let cool.

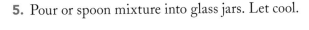

Evening Primrose Face Cream for Acne

When applying this cream, use your fingers to lightly massage your face. It will help the mixture penetrate the skin so it can get to work clearing up acne.

Best for: Acne-prone skin on the face

Tip: Use a large, sharp sewing needle to pierce the evening primrose oil capsules so you can squeeze out the contents. The bigger the hole, the faster the process will go.

Note: Exact measurements are important when you're making skin- and hair-care products. Turn to page 17 for how-tos.

20	capsules (each 500 mg) evening primrose oil	20
0.35 oz	jojoba oil	10 g
0.28 oz	cocoa butter	8 g
0.2 oz	Lanette wax (see box, page 15)	6 g
6 oz	witch hazel	170 g
2	pinches citric acid powder (see box, page 27)	2
2	pinches ascorbic acid powder	2
5	drops bergamot essential oil	5
5	drops tea tree essential oil	5

1. Using a large needle, pierce evening primrose oil capsules and squeeze the contents into a saucepan (see tip, at left). Add jojoba oil, cocoa butter and Lanette wax. Heat over low heat just until ingredients are completely melted. Remove from heat and keep warm.

2. Pour witch hazel into a separate saucepan. Heat until lukewarm. Using a wooden spoon, stir in citric acid and ascorbic acid until dissolved.

3. Stir witch hazel mixture into oil mixture. Using a hand mixer, beat at low speed for 1 to 2 minutes. Let stand for 10 minutes.

4. Stir in bergamot and tea tree essential oils. Using a hand mixer, beat at high speed for 1 minute.

5. Pour or spoon mixture into glass jars. Let cool.

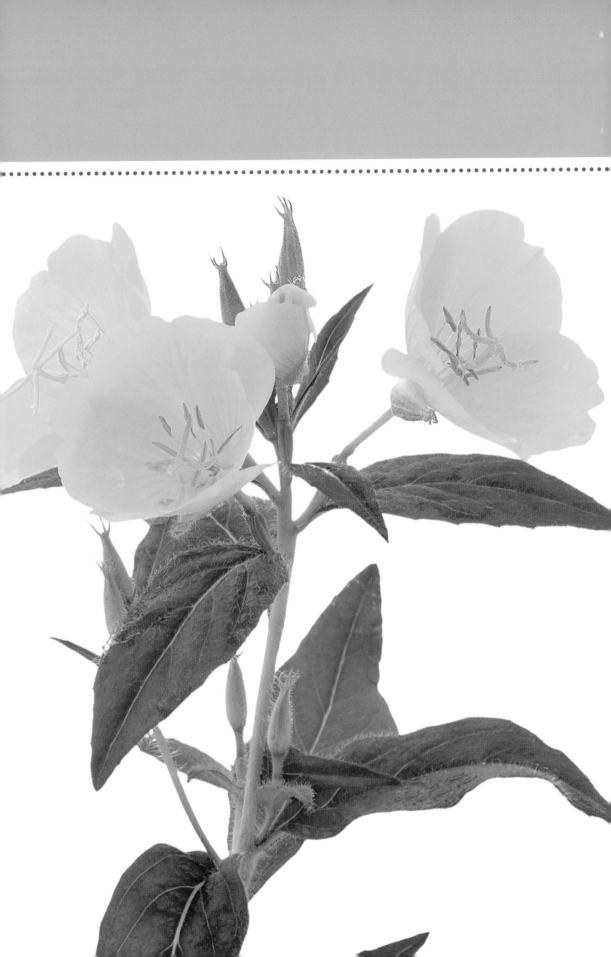

Evening Primrose Body Cream for Acne

Acne isn't something that affects just the face. It can also spread to the chest, upper arms and back, with painful results. This cream will treat the underlying cause while soothing and improving the skin.

Best for: Acne-prone skin on the back, arms and chest

Tip: Use a large, sharp sewing needle to pierce the evening primrose oil capsules so you can squeeze out the contents. The bigger the hole, the faster the process will go.

Note: Exact measurements are important when you're making skin- and hair-care products. Turn to page 17 for how-tos.

25	capsules (each 500 mg) evening primrose oil	25
0.4 oz	Lanette wax (see box, page 15)	12 g
0.35 oz	jojoba oil	10 g
0.18 oz	cocoa butter	5 g
12.7 oz	mineral water	360 g
4	pinches citric acid powder (see box, page 27)	4
4	pinches ascorbic acid powder	4
10	drops cypress essential oil	10
10	drops tea tree essential oil	10

1. Using a large needle, pierce evening primrose oil capsules and squeeze the contents into a saucepan (see tip, at left). Add Lanette wax, jojoba oil and cocoa butter. Heat over low heat just until ingredients are completely melted. Remove from heat and keep warm.

2. Pour mineral water into a separate saucepan. Heat until lukewarm. Using a wooden spoon, stir in citric acid and ascorbic acid until dissolved.

3. Stir mineral water mixture into oil mixture. Using a hand mixer, beat at low speed for 1 to 2 minutes. Let stand for 10 minutes.

4. Stir in cypress and tea tree essential oils. Using a hand mixer, beat at high speed for 1 minute.

5. Pour or spoon mixture into glass jars. Let cool.

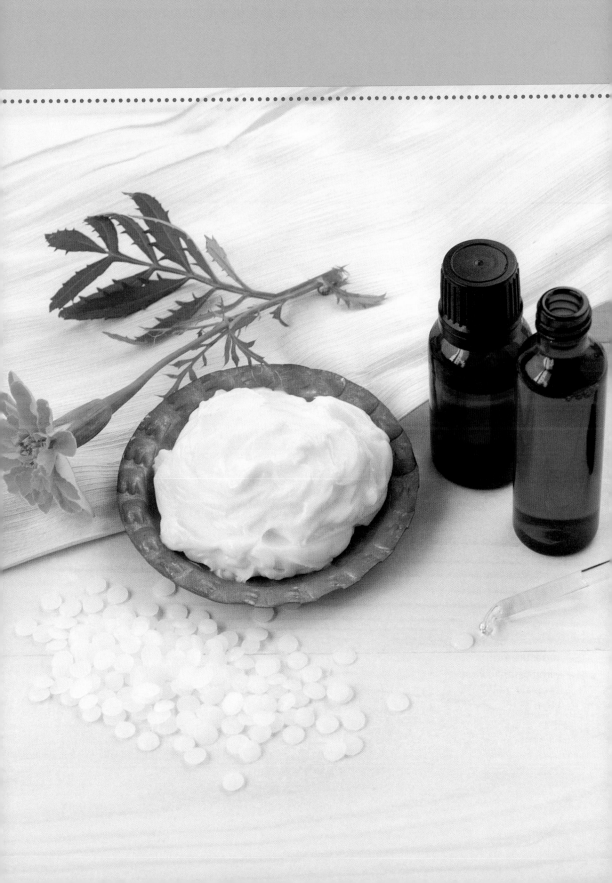

Evening Primrose Nourishing Oil

Vetiver and chamomile give this rich oil a lovely scent. To apply it, place a few drops on your fingertips and gently spread over your face and neck.

Best for: Dry skin

Tip: Store the finished oil away from light to keep its healing properties intact. This is a smart policy for all homemade oils.

Note: Exact measurements are important when you're making skin- and hair-care products. Turn to page 17 for how-tos.

10	capsules (each 500 mg) evening primrose oil	10
0.35 oz	sweet almond oil	10 g
5	drops vetiver essential oil	5
5	drops chamomile essential oil (see tip, below)	5

1. Using a large needle, pierce evening primrose oil capsules and squeeze the contents into a small glass bottle (see tip, opposite). Add sweet almond oil, and vetiver and chamomile essential oils. Seal tightly.

2. Shake to combine.

Tip: You'll often find two types of chamomile essential oil at cosmetic-supply stores: German and Roman. They come from different strains of the chamomile plant, but both are soothing additions to homemade skin- and hair-care products.

Using Evening Primrose Oil to Treat Raynaud's Disease

Pure evening primrose oil is a simple, effective tool you can use to stimulate the cool, reddened skin associated with this disease. Pierce several evening primrose capsules and squeeze out the oil, then massage it over the affected areas, such as the toes, fingers, ears and nose.

Evening Primrose Injury-Healing Oil

This is a small-batch treatment for all sorts of injuries. Gently massage the oil into the skin immediately after preparing it.

Best for: Strains, sprains and muscle tears

Tip: Use a large, sharp sewing needle to pierce the evening primrose oil capsules so you can squeeze out the contents. The bigger the hole, the faster the process will go.

Caution: Do not use rosemary essential oil if you have epilepsy or high blood pressure.

10	capsules (each 500 mg) evening primrose oil	10
5	drops rosemary essential oil (see caution, at left)	5
5	drops ginger essential oil	5

1. Using a large needle, pierce evening primrose oil capsules and squeeze the contents into a small bowl (see tip, at left). Add rosemary and ginger essential oils.

2. Stir until well combined. Use immediately.

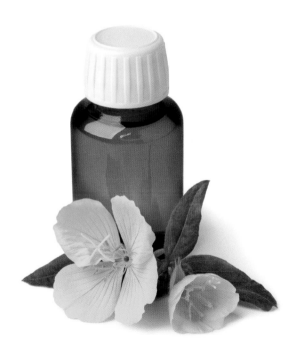

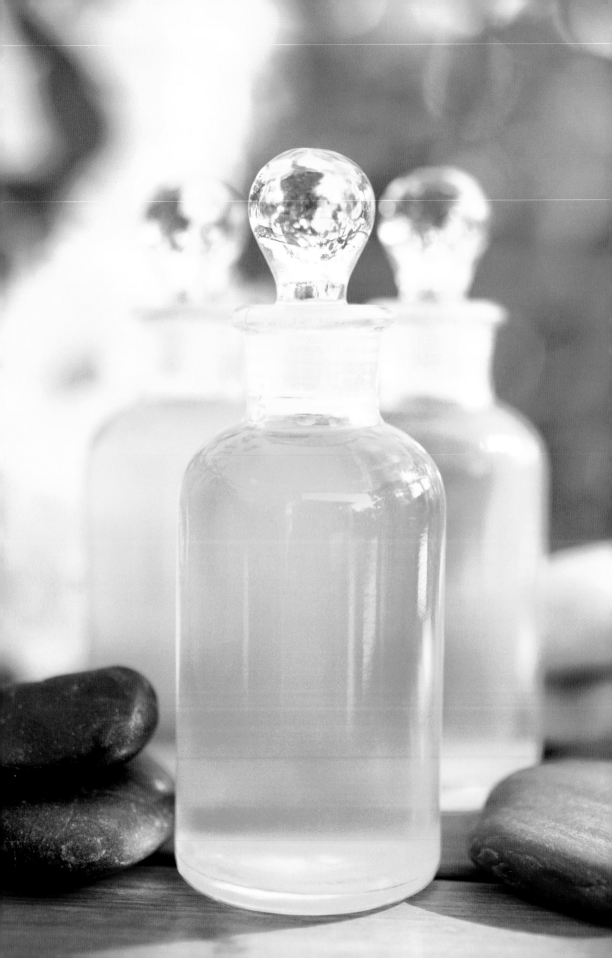

Babassu Oil

Babassu oil is suitable for all skin types.
Its greatest strength is that it is a
powerful firming agent.

The use of babassu oil in food and cosmetics in Latin America dates back to the Mayan period. The babassu palm tree is grown extensively in Brazil, and the seeds are cold pressed to extract this rich oil. To prevent deforestation and promote conservation of the trees, women have formed cooperatives in order to harvest the oil responsibly. They sell the oil and feed their families from the proceeds. In recent years, the Brazilian government has created laws that guarantee the women's right to harvest the babassu nut, even on private property.

Babassu oil is rich in fatty acids, including lauric, myristic, palmitic, caprylic and stearic acids. It has a balanced ratio of fatty acids to tocotrienols to phytosterols. Tocotrienols are part of the vitamin E family, and are more effective antioxidants than tocopherols, a more familiar form of vitamin E. Phytosterols enhance the protective barrier on the skin, delay aging and protect skin from damaging ultraviolet rays.

Babassu oil is very liquid and less greasy than other oils. It rapidly penetrates the inner dermis layer of the skin, and doesn't leave a slick, oily feel behind. It is an excellent moisturizer and works well for all skin types, but is especially well suited to naturally oily skin. It protects the hair and revitalizes dry ends, as well.

Babassu and Soy Moisturizing Face Cream

Just a hint of tea tree and rosemary essential oils gives this cream a refreshing, exhilarating scent.

Best for: Oily skin

Tip: Look for chunks or blocks of pure cocoa butter at cosmetic-supply stores. If you're using a large amount in a recipe, chop it up before adding it to the saucepan so it will melt more quickly.

Note: Exact measurements are important when you're making skin- and hair-care products. Turn to page 17 for how-tos.

Caution: Do not use rosemary essential oil if you have epilepsy or high blood pressure.

0.2 oz	Lanette wax (see box, page 15)	6 g
0.18 oz	babassu oil	5 g
0.18 oz	soybean oil	5 g
0.15 oz	cocoa butter (see tip, at left)	4 g
6.3 oz	witch hazel	180 g
2	pinches citric acid powder (see box, page 27)	2
2	pinches ascorbic acid powder	2
4	drops tea tree essential oil	4
4	drops rosemary essential oil (see caution, at left)	4

1. Combine Lanette wax, babassu oil, soybean oil and cocoa butter in a saucepan. Heat over low heat just until ingredients are completely melted. Remove from heat and keep warm.

2. Pour witch hazel into a separate saucepan. Heat until lukewarm. Using a wooden spoon, stir in citric acid and ascorbic acid until dissolved.

3. Stir witch hazel mixture into oil mixture. Using a hand mixer, beat at low speed for 1 to 2 minutes. Let stand for 10 minutes.

4. Stir in tea tree and rosemary essential oils. Using a hand mixer, beat at high speed for 1 minute.

5. Pour or spoon mixture into glass jars. Let cool.

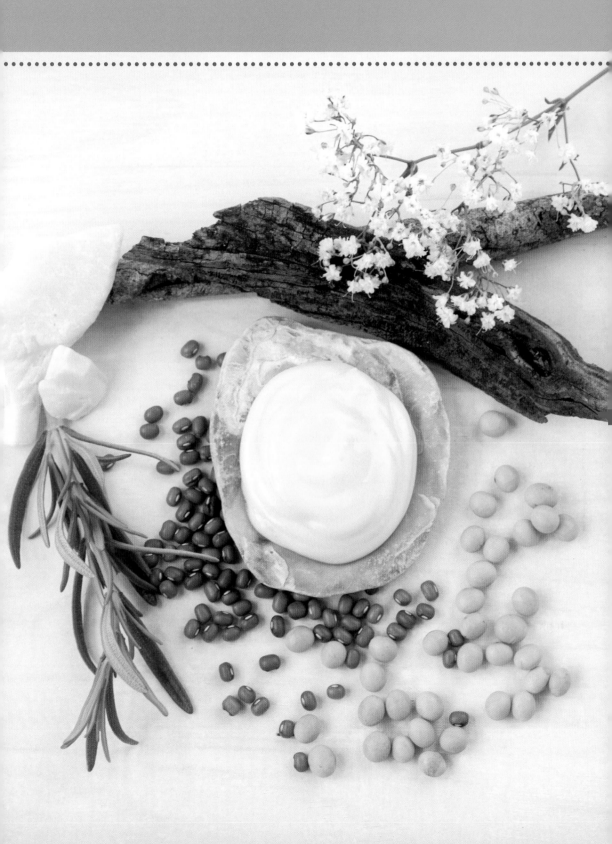

Babassu Anti-Wrinkle Moisturizing Face Cream

Oily skin needs proper nutrition. This cream leaves skin smooth and well nourished, without a greasy feel.

Best for: Oily skin

Tips: Orange flower water is also called orange blossom water. It's easy to find in Middle Eastern grocery stores and some well-stocked supermarkets, where it's sold for use in cooking.

The essential oils you use for skin- and hair-care products must be 100% pure. Don't use synthetic scents or oils, or essences used in fragrance burners or lamp rings.

Note: Exact measurements are important when you're making skin- and hair-care products. Turn to page 17 for how-tos.

0.2 oz	Lanette wax (see box, page 15)	6 g
0.18 oz	babassu oil	5 g
0.18 oz	St. John's wort oil	5 g
0.18 oz	jojoba oil	5 g
0.07 oz	cocoa butter	2 g
6.2 oz	orange flower water (see tips, at left)	175 g
2	pinches citric acid powder (see box, page 27)	2
2	pinches ascorbic acid powder	2
15	drops cedar essential oil (see tips, at left)	15

1. Combine Lanette wax, babassu oil, St. John's wort oil, jojoba oil and cocoa butter in a saucepan. Heat over low heat just until ingredients are completely melted. Remove from heat and keep warm.

2. Pour orange flower water into a separate saucepan. Heat until lukewarm. Using a wooden spoon, stir in citric acid and ascorbic acid until dissolved.

3. Stir orange flower water mixture into oil mixture. Using a hand mixer, beat at low speed for 1 to 2 minutes. Let stand for 10 minutes.

4. Stir in cedar essential oil. Using a hand mixer, beat at high speed for 1 minute.

5. Pour or spoon mixture into glass jars. Let cool.

Babassu Nourishing Face Cream

Oily skin needs moisturizing just like dry skin, but it requires different ingredients. This cream is easily absorbed and, thanks to the babassu oil, is especially suited to oily skin.

Best for: Oily skin

Tip: Citronella essential oil has a strong lemongrass-like aroma. It's often used in perfumes, and is a natural insect repellent.

Note: Exact measurements are important when you're making skin- and hair-care products. Turn to page 17 for how-tos.

0.35 oz	babassu oil	10 g
0.2 oz	Lanette wax (see box, page 15)	6 g
0.18 oz	cocoa butter	5 g
6 oz	mineral water	170 g
2	pinches citric acid powder (see box, page 27)	2
2	pinches ascorbic acid powder	2
0.35 oz	liquid glycerin	10 g
10	drops citronella essential oil (see tip, at left)	10

1. Combine babassu oil, Lanette wax and cocoa butter in a saucepan. Heat over low heat just until ingredients are completely melted. Remove from heat and keep warm.

2. Pour mineral water into a separate saucepan. Heat until lukewarm. Using a wooden spoon, stir in citric acid and ascorbic acid until dissolved.

3. Stir mineral water mixture into oil mixture. Using a hand mixer, beat at low speed for 1 to 2 minutes. Let stand for 10 minutes.

4. Stir in glycerin and citronella essential oil. Using a hand mixer, beat at high speed for 1 minute.

5. Pour or spoon mixture into glass jars. Let cool.

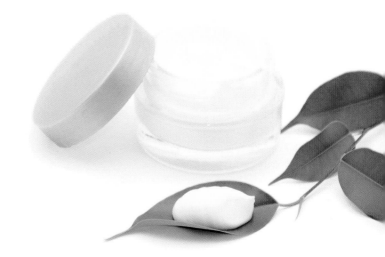

Babassu Moisturizing Body Cream

Contrary to popular belief, oily skin can be deeply dehydrated, despite its appearance. This cream is the perfect remedy, and it smells heavenly.

Best for: Oily skin

Tips: Rose water is frequently used in Middle Eastern and Mediterranean cooking. Look for it in Middle Eastern grocery stores and some well-stocked supermarkets.

Liquid glycerin is a moisturizing ingredient often included in cosmetics, soaps, shampoos and creams. You'll find small bottles of it at drugstores, but cosmetic-supply stores sell larger bulk amounts.

Note: Exact measurements are important when you're making skin- and hair-care products. Turn to page 17 for how-tos.

0.5 oz	babassu oil	15 g
0.4 oz	Lanette wax (see box, page 15)	12 g
0.18 oz	coconut oil	5 g
12.7 oz	rose water (see tips, at left)	360 g
4	pinches citric acid powder (see box, page 27)	4
4	pinches ascorbic acid powder	4
0.35 oz	liquid glycerin (see tips, at left)	10 g
10	drops cypress essential oil	10
10	drops lemon essential oil	10

1. Combine babassu oil, Lanette wax and coconut oil in a saucepan. Heat over low heat just until ingredients are completely melted. Remove from heat and keep warm.

2. Pour rose water into a separate saucepan. Heat until lukewarm. Using a wooden spoon, stir in citric acid and ascorbic acid until dissolved.

3. Stir rose water mixture into oil mixture. Using a hand mixer, beat at low speed for 1 to 2 minutes. Let stand for 10 minutes.

4. Stir in glycerin, and cypress and lemon essential oils. Using a hand mixer, beat at high speed for 1 minute.

5. Pour or spoon mixture into glass jars. Let cool.

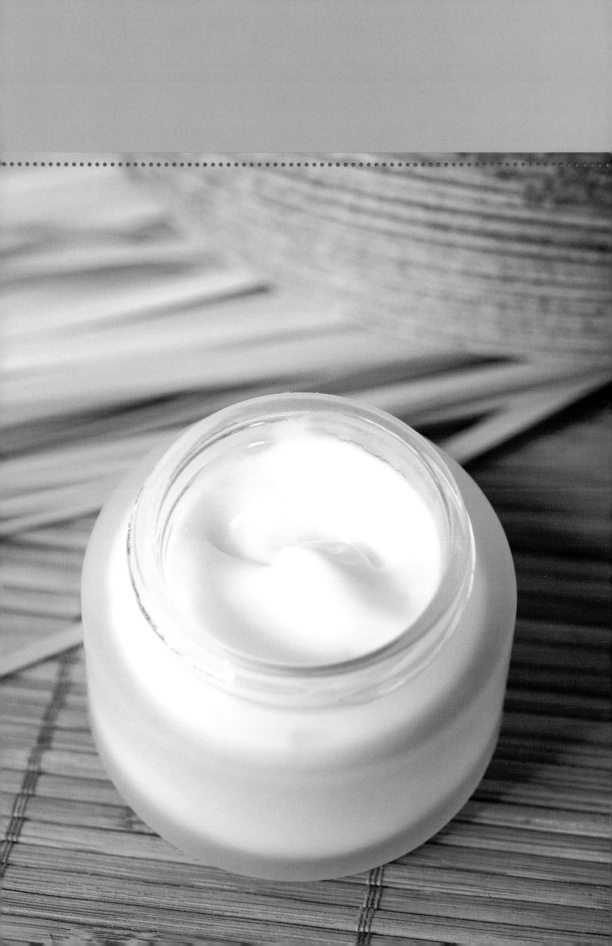

Babassu Exfoliating Scrub

2.3 oz	fine sea salt	65 g
0.9 oz	babassu oil	25 g
7	drops grapefruit essential oil	7

1. Combine sea salt, babassu oil and grapefruit essential oil in a bowl.

2. Using a wooden spoon, stir until ingredients are well combined. Use immediately.

This scrub moisturizes the skin so well, there's no need to apply body cream after you're done. Just wash and go!

Best for: Oily skin

Tip: Apply to the face and body using a gentle circular motion. After you're done, wash the scrub off completely with water and mild soap. Repeat once a week.

Note: Exact measurements are important when you're making skin- and hair-care products. Turn to page 17 for how-tos.

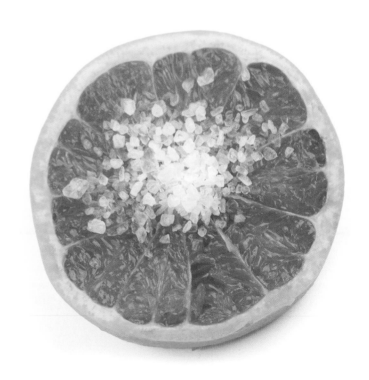

Babassu Sunscreen

This cream is excellent for sun protection most of the year. In the summer, when the sun's rays are stronger, it is better suited to people who tan easily (fair-skinned people should use a more protective alternative).

Best for: All skin types

Tip: The essential oils you use for skin- and hair-care products must be 100% pure. Don't use synthetic scents or oils, or essences used in fragrance burners or lamp rings.

Note: Exact measurements are important when you're making skin- and hair-care products. Turn to page 17 for how-tos.

0.4 oz	Lanette wax (see box, page 15)	12 g
0.35 oz	babassu oil	10 g
0.35 oz	avocado oil	10 g
0.35 oz	walnut oil	10 g
12.5 oz	rose water	355 g
4	pinches citric acid powder (see box, page 27)	4
4	pinches ascorbic acid powder	4
0.04 oz	carrot seed essential oil (see tip, at left)	1 g

1. Combine Lanette wax, babassu oil, avocado oil and walnut oil in a saucepan. Heat over low heat just until ingredients are completely melted. Remove from heat and keep warm.

2. Pour rose water into a separate saucepan. Heat until lukewarm. Using a wooden spoon, stir in citric acid and ascorbic acid until dissolved.

3. Stir rose water mixture into oil mixture. Using a hand mixer, beat at low speed for 1 to 2 minutes. Let stand for 10 minutes.

4. Stir in carrot seed essential oil. Using a hand mixer, beat at high speed for 1 minute.

5. Pour or spoon mixture into glass jars. Let cool.

Babassu and Green Clay Facial Mask

Clay purifies the skin, so it's excellent in a mask. Use this one to remove impurities and leave skin feeling incredibly soft.

Best for: Oily skin

Tip: Green clay is often added to facial masks and treatments, and is thought to stimulate blood flow to injured areas and speed up the healing process. Look for it in powdered form at cosmetic-supply stores.

Note: Exact measurements are important when you're making skin- and hair-care products. Turn to page 17 for how-tos.

0.7 oz	green clay (see tip, at left)	20 g
0.35 oz	babassu oil	10 g
3	drops sandalwood essential oil	3

1. Combine green clay, babassu oil and sandalwood essential oil in a bowl.
2. Using a wooden spoon, stir well until ingredients are combined. Use immediately.

Tip: Use a thick brush to apply the mask to the face and neck. Let it dry for 10 minutes, then wash it off with cold water. Don't use warm or hot water, because the clay may react and cause a rash.

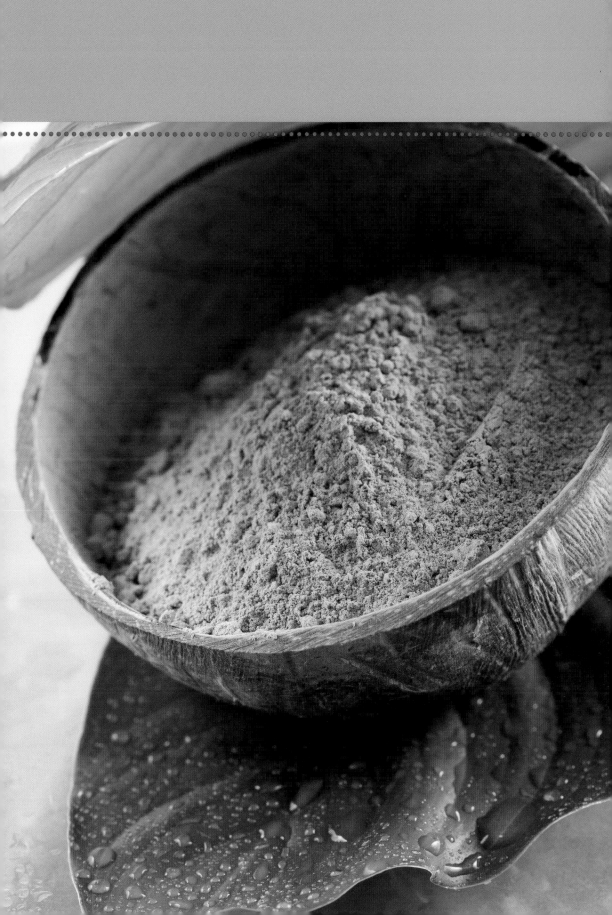

Babassu and Chamomile Shampoo

Best for:
Normal hair

Tips: Coco betaine (short for cocamido-propyl betaine) is a surfactant made from coconut oil and gives shampoos their cleaning power and lather. It's easy to find at cosmetic-supply stores.

You'll often find two types of chamomile essential oil at cosmetic-supply stores: German and Roman. They come from different strains of the chamomile plant, but both are soothing additions to homemade skin- and hair-care products.

2 tbsp	fresh or dried chamomile flowers	30 mL
4.9 oz	mineral water	140 g
4.2 oz	coco betaine (see tips, at left)	120 g
0.07 oz	babassu oil	2 g
10	drops chamomile essential oil (see tips, at left)	10

1. Place chamomile flowers in a heatproof bowl. In a saucepan, bring mineral water to a boil. Pour boiling mineral water over chamomile flowers. Cover and let steep for 10 minutes.

2. Using a fine-mesh sieve lined with cheesecloth, strain the chamomile infusion into a clean bowl. Let cool completely.

3. Pour chamomile infusion, coco betaine, babassu oil and chamomile essential oil into a bottle. Seal tightly. Shake gently to combine.

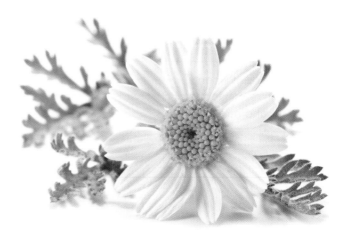

Babassu Body Oil

The most convenient way to apply this oil is to use a small bottle with a roll-on top. Once the bottle is empty, it can be washed and reused.

Best for: All skin types

Tip: Petitgrain essential oil is made from the leaves and twigs of the bitter orange tree. It has a beautiful scent that is different from the scents of orange and neroli essential oils, which are made from other parts of the tree. Petitgrain essential oil is often an ingredient in perfumes.

Note: Exact measurements are important when you're making skin- and hair-care products. Turn to page 17 for how-tos.

| 3.5 oz | babassu oil | 100 g |
| 0.07 oz | petitgrain essential oil (see tip, at left) | 2 g |

1. Pour babassu oil and petitgrain essential oil into a small glass bottle. Seal tightly.
2. Shake to combine.

Babassu Oil Soothes Joint Pain

Babassu oil can be used for all types of massages, on its own or combined with other base or essential oils. It has anti-inflammatory properties, so it makes a terrific massage oil — without any additions — for treating sore joints.

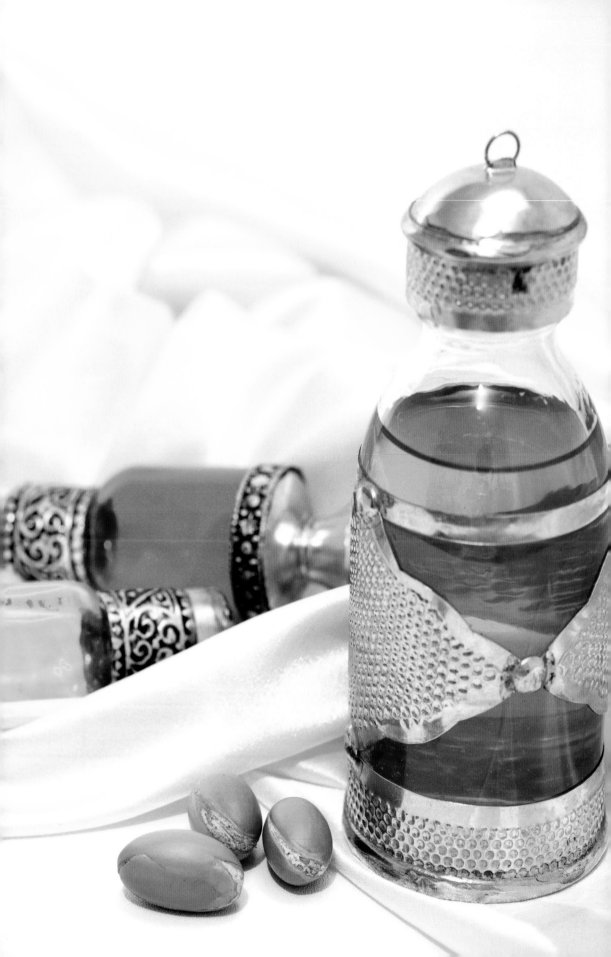

Argan Oil

Argan oil is one of the most highly recommended oils for the treatment of skin blemishes.

This incredible oil is pressed from the seeds of the fruit of the argan tree *(Argania spinosa),* which grows only in the semiarid regions of southwestern Morocco. It is believed that this magnificent tree came into existence as many as 80,000 years ago. Its roots can reach down 100 feet (30 m) in search of water.

The argan tree has been used as a source of food for centuries. To make an edible oil for cooking, argan seeds are lightly roasted, then cold pressed. It takes about 65 lbs (29.5 kg) of seeds to produce 4 cups (1 L) of argan oil. To make an oil for use in skin- and hair-care formulas, argan seeds are cold pressed, but the roasting step is skipped.

Argan oil contains 48% omega-9 oleic acid and 32% omega-6 linoleic acid. It has one of the highest levels of tocopherols (alpha-, gamma- and delta-tocopherols) of any oil. It also contains spinasterol and schottenol, two rare phytosterols that are found in no other oils.

Argan oil is an excellent ingredient in cooking, but it is even better in skin- and hair-care products. It combats dry skin and hair, prevents stretch marks, reduces age spots and is a potent cell regenerator, making it beneficial for treating wrinkles. Whether used alone or mixed with essential oils, argan oil is highly recommended for use in all types of massage.

Argan Regenerating Face Cream

Try this cream to repair damaged skin with premature wrinkles or skin that has been exposed to harsh weather.

Best for: Damaged or wrinkled skin

Tips: Pure shea butter comes in chunks, like cocoa butter, at cosmetic-supply stores. Break or chop it up before adding it to the saucepan so that it melts quickly and easily.

Lanolin is a waxy natural moisturizer derived from sheep's wool. It has long been used as a softening and moisturizing agent, especially in hand creams. You can find jars of it at cosmetic-supply stores. It has a distinctive, earthy aroma, and a little goes a long way.

0.5 oz	argan oil	15 g
0.2 oz	Lanette wax (see box, page 15)	6 g
0.15 oz	shea butter (see tips, at left)	4 g
0.15 oz	beeswax (see tip, below)	4 g
0.07 oz	wheat germ oil (see tip, page 96)	2 g
0.07 oz	lanolin (see tips, at left)	2 g
5.5 oz	orange flower water	155 g
2	pinches citric acid powder (see box, page 27)	2
2	pinches ascorbic acid powder	2
0.18 oz	rose hip seed oil	5 g
20	drops myrrh essential oil	20

1. Combine argan oil, Lanette wax, shea butter, beeswax, wheat germ oil and lanolin in a saucepan. Heat over low heat just until ingredients are completely melted. Remove from heat and keep warm.

2. Pour orange flower water into a separate saucepan. Heat until lukewarm. Using a wooden spoon, stir in citric acid and ascorbic acid until dissolved.

3. Stir orange flower water mixture into oil mixture. Using a hand mixer, beat at low speed for 1 to 2 minutes. Let stand for 10 minutes.

4. Stir in rose hip seed oil and myrrh essential oil. Using a hand mixer, beat at high speed for 1 minute.

5. Pour or spoon mixture into glass jars. Let cool.

Tip: Look for 100% pure beeswax that has been minimally processed. It is often sold in bulk, in chunks; if the recipe calls for a large amount, grate the wax so it will melt quickly and smoothly. Alternatively, you can buy beeswax that has been formed into pearls, which are easy to measure and melt quickly.

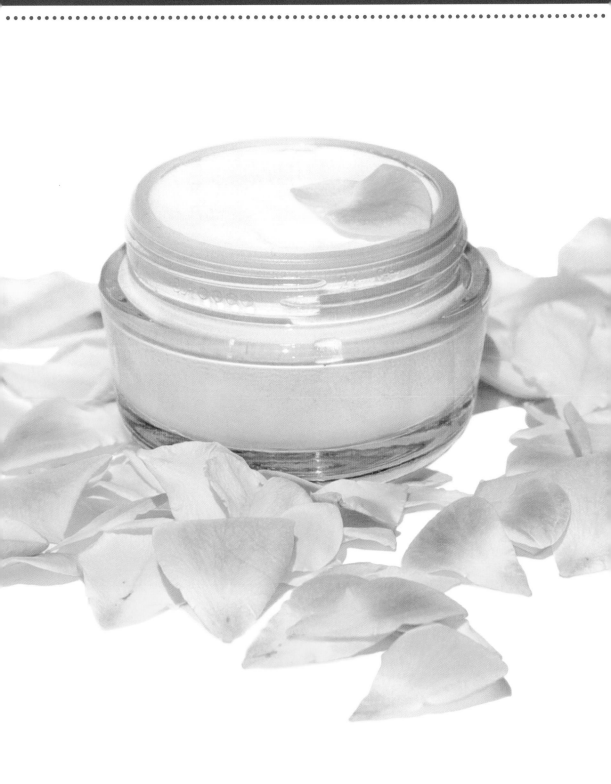

Argan Anti–Stretch Mark Cream

Stretch marks can form following an increase or decrease in body weight, and pregnant women are particularly prone to them. Regular application of this cream will help prevent them.

Best for: Areas prone to stretch marks, such as the belly, thighs and buttocks

Tips: Look for chunks or blocks of pure cocoa butter at cosmetic-supply stores. If you're using a large amount in a recipe, chop it up before adding it to the saucepan so it will melt more quickly.

Rose water is often used in Middle Eastern and Mediterranean cooking. Look for it in Middle Eastern grocery stores and some well-stocked supermarkets.

2.1 oz	argan oil	60 g
0.35 oz	cocoa butter (see tips, at left)	10 g
0.2 oz	Lanette wax (see box, page 15)	6 g
0.15 oz	beeswax	4 g
4.2 oz	rose water (see tips, at left)	120 g
2	pinches citric acid powder (see box, page 27)	2
2	pinches ascorbic acid powder	2

1. Combine argan oil, cocoa butter, Lanette wax and beeswax in a saucepan. Heat over low heat just until ingredients are completely melted. Remove from heat and keep warm.

2. Pour rose water into a separate saucepan. Heat until lukewarm. Using a wooden spoon, stir in citric acid and ascorbic acid until dissolved.

3. Stir rose water mixture into oil mixture. Using a hand mixer, beat at low speed for 1 to 2 minutes. Let stand for 10 minutes.

4. Using a hand mixer, beat at high speed for 1 minute.

5. Pour or spoon mixture into glass jars. Let cool.

Argan Anti-Acne Face Cream

Soothe and protect acne-prone skin with this lovely cream. Rub gently as you apply it, to avoid irritating sore spots.

Best for: Acne-prone skin

Tip: Citronella essential oil has a strong lemongrass-like aroma. It's often used in perfumes, and is a natural insect repellent.

Note: Exact measurements are important when you're making skin- and hair-care products. Turn to page 17 for how-tos.

0.35 oz	argan oil	10 g
0.2 oz	Lanette wax (see box, page 15)	6 g
0.15 oz	jojoba oil	4 g
6.3 oz	mineral water	180 g
2	pinches citric acid powder (see box, page 27)	2
2	pinches ascorbic acid powder	2
10	drops citronella essential oil (see tip, at left)	10
10	drops cypress essential oil	10
4	drops bergamot essential oil	4

1. Combine argan oil, Lanette wax and jojoba oil in a saucepan. Heat over low heat just until ingredients are completely melted. Remove from heat and keep warm.

2. Pour mineral water into a separate saucepan. Heat until lukewarm. Using a wooden spoon, stir in citric acid and ascorbic acid until dissolved.

3. Stir mineral water mixture into oil mixture. Using a hand mixer, beat at low speed for 1 to 2 minutes. Let stand for 10 minutes.

4. Stir in citronella, cypress and bergamot essential oils. Using a hand mixer, beat at high speed for 1 minute.

5. Pour or spoon mixture into glass jars. Let cool.

Vitamin-Rich Argan After-Sun Cream

Apply a generous amount of this rich cream to your face and body after exposure to the sun at the beach or pool. It will keep hard-working skin supple.

Best for: All skin types

Tips: Liquid glycerin is a moisturizing ingredient often included in cosmetics, soaps, shampoos and creams. You'll find small bottles of it at drugstores, but cosmetic-supply stores sell larger bulk amounts.

Look for pure vitamins A and E in liquid form at cosmetic-supply stores. They're also easy to buy online.

Note: Exact measurements are important when you're making skin- and hair-care products. Turn to page 17 for how-tos.

0.7 oz	argan oil	20 g
0.4 oz	Lanette wax (see box, page 15)	12 g
0.18 oz	sesame oil	5 g
0.18 oz	sunflower oil	5 g
0.18 oz	cocoa butter	5 g
12 oz	rose water	340 g
0.35 oz	liquid glycerin (see tips, at left)	10 g
0.1 oz	pure vitamin A (see tips, at left)	3 g
0.1 oz	pure vitamin E	3 g

1. Combine argan oil, Lanette wax, sesame oil, sunflower oil and cocoa butter in a saucepan. Heat over low heat just until ingredients are completely melted. Remove from heat and keep warm.

2. Pour rose water into a separate saucepan. Heat just until lukewarm.

3. Stir rose water into oil mixture. Using a hand mixer, beat at low speed for 1 to 2 minutes. Let stand for 10 minutes.

4. Stir in glycerin, and vitamins A and E. Using a hand mixer, beat at high speed for 1 minute.

5. Pour or spoon mixture into glass jars. Let cool.

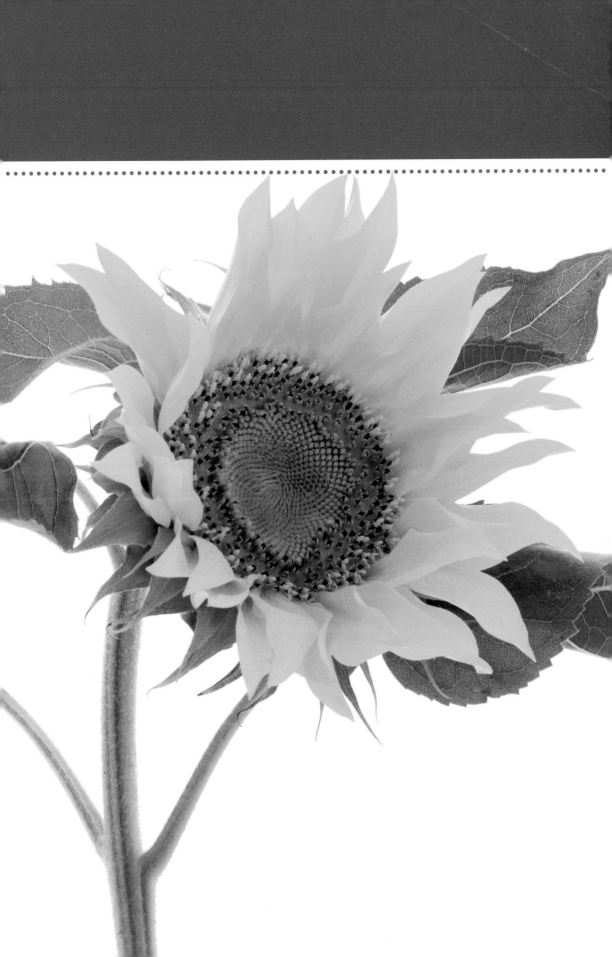

Argan Eye Cream

This cream is specially designed to reduce puffy skin under the eyes and on the eyelids. Spread it around the eye area, massaging with gentle circular motions.

Best for: Under-eye bags and puffy eyes

Note: Exact measurements are important when you're making skin- and hair-care products. Turn to page 17 for how-tos.

0.35 oz	argan oil	10 g
0.18 oz	flaxseed oil	5 g
0.1 oz	Lanette wax (see box, page 15)	3 g
2.9 oz	witch hazel	82 g
1	pinch ascorbic acid powder (see box, page 27)	1
3	drops myrrh essential oil	3

1. Combine argan oil, flaxseed oil and Lanette wax in a saucepan. Heat over low heat just until ingredients are completely melted. Remove from heat and keep warm.

2. Pour witch hazel into a separate saucepan. Heat until lukewarm. Using a wooden spoon, stir in ascorbic acid until dissolved.

3. Stir witch hazel mixture into oil mixture. Using a hand mixer, beat at low speed for 1 to 2 minutes. Let stand for 10 minutes.

4. Stir in myrrh essential oil. Using a hand mixer, beat at high speed for 1 minute.

5. Pour or spoon mixture into glass jars. Let cool.

Protect Your Hair with Argan Oil

Argan oil is an ideal tool for keeping hair healthy and beautiful. This simple treatment will protect your tresses from the damaging effects of sun, sea and chlorine. Place a few drops of argan oil in the palms of your hands and rub it through your hair, from the roots to the ends. Let stand for 1 hour. Shampoo your hair as usual, rinsing well. Enjoy the silky results.

Argan Hand Cream

Used regularly,
this cream
will keep your
hands perfectly
moisturized.

Best for: Dry hands

Tips: Look for
chunks or blocks of
pure cocoa butter
at cosmetic-supply
stores. If you're using
a large amount in a
recipe, chop it up
before adding it to
the saucepan so it will
melt more quickly.

Store essential oils
in a cool, dark place.
Light exposure
can diminish their
healing properties.

Note: Exact
measurements are
important when
you're making
skin- and hair-care
products. Turn to
page 17 for how-tos.

0.7 oz	argan oil	20 g
0.2 oz	Lanette wax (see box, page 15)	6 g
0.18 oz	cocoa butter (see tips, at left)	5 g
5.5 oz	mineral water	155 g
2	pinches citric acid powder (see box, page 27)	2
2	pinches ascorbic acid powder	2
0.18 oz	liquid glycerin	5 g
10	drops geranium essential oil (see tips, at left)	10

1. Combine argan oil, Lanette wax and cocoa butter in a saucepan. Heat over low heat just until ingredients are completely melted. Remove from heat and keep warm.

2. Pour mineral water into a separate saucepan. Heat until lukewarm. Using a wooden spoon, stir in citric acid and ascorbic acid until dissolved.

3. Stir mineral water mixture into oil mixture. Using a hand mixer, beat at low speed for 1 to 2 minutes. Let stand for 10 minutes.

4. Stir in glycerin and geranium essential oil. Using a hand mixer, beat at high speed for 1 minute.

5. Pour or spoon mixture into glass jars. Let cool.

Argan Oil and Lemon Nail Soak

In a small bowl, mix equal parts lemon juice and argan oil. Soak your nails in this mixture for 20 minutes once a week. You'll have strong, well-conditioned nails you can count on.

Argan Foot Cream

When thick dry skin, calluses and cracks make your feet sore and tired, reach for this cream. It will moisturize and protect the skin, encouraging it to heal.

Best for: Very dry feet and cracked heels

Tip: Look for 100% pure beeswax that has been minimally processed. It is often sold in bulk, in chunks; if the recipe calls for a large amount, grate the wax so it will melt quickly and smoothly. Alternatively, you can buy beeswax that has been formed into pearls, which are easy to measure and melt quickly.

Caution: Do not use rosemary essential oil if you have epilepsy or high blood pressure.

0.35 oz	argan oil	10 g
0.35 oz	beeswax (see tip, at left)	10 g
0.35 oz	lanolin (see tip, below)	10 g
0.2 oz	Lanette wax (see box, page 15)	6 g
0.18 oz	cocoa butter	5 g
5.6 oz	mineral water	160 g
2	pinches citric acid powder (see box, page 27)	2
2	pinches ascorbic acid powder	2
10	drops tea tree essential oil	10
10	drops rosemary essential oil (see caution, at left)	10

1. Combine argan oil, beeswax, lanolin, Lanette wax and cocoa butter in a saucepan. Heat over low heat just until ingredients are completely melted. Remove from heat and keep warm.

2. Pour mineral water into a separate saucepan. Heat until lukewarm. Using a wooden spoon, stir in citric acid and ascorbic acid until dissolved.

3. Stir mineral water mixture into oil mixture. Using a hand mixer, beat at low speed for 1 to 2 minutes. Let stand for 10 minutes.

4. Stir in tea tree and rosemary essential oils. Using a hand mixer, beat at high speed for 1 minute.

5. Pour or spoon mixture into glass jars. Let cool.

Tip: Lanolin is a waxy natural moisturizer derived from sheep's wool. It has long been used as a softening and moisturizing agent, especially in hand and foot creams. You can find jars of it at cosmetic-supply stores. It has a distinctive, earthy aroma, and a little goes a long way.

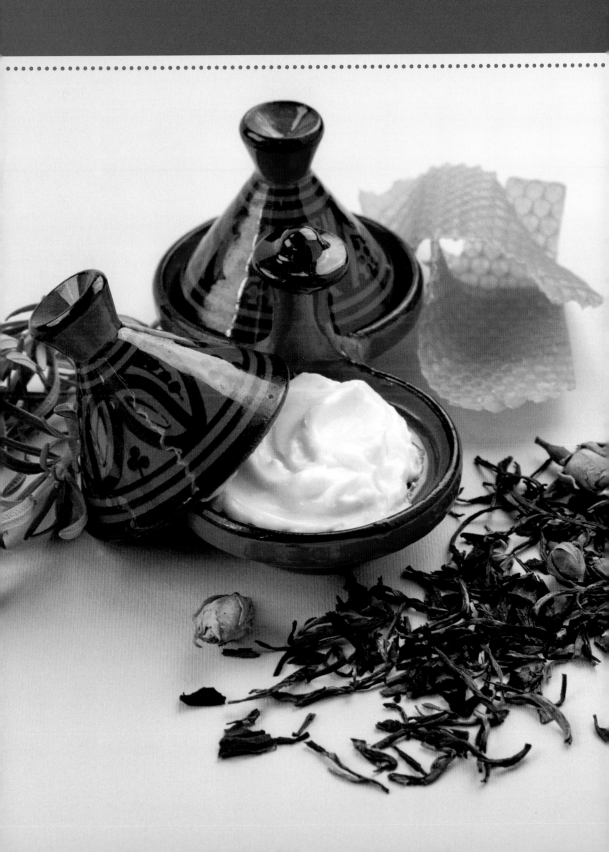

Argan Healing Oil

This very simple mixture is the key to healing sore, red and wounded skin. The lavender oil is soothing for both body and mind.

Best for: Sores, chilblains and burns

0.35 oz	argan oil	10 g
1	drop lavender essential oil	1

1. Pour argan oil and lavender essential oil into a small glass bottle. Seal tightly.
2. Shake to combine.

Tip: Gently apply a couple of drops of the oil to the affected area. To treat chilblains, massage the area for a few minutes until the oil is absorbed.

Argan Relaxing Massage Oil

This oil is ideal to use when giving a soothing, relaxing full-body massage. The subtle aroma of ylang-ylang contributes to the pleasure of the experience.

Best for: All skin types

0.7 oz	argan oil	20 g
10	drops ylang-ylang essential oil	10

1. Pour argan oil and ylang-ylang essential oil into a small glass bottle. Seal tightly.
2. Shake to combine.

Argan Blemish-Fighting Oil

Once a day, use a cotton ball to spread this simple oil over the affected area. Then sit back and watch those blemishes disappear!

Best for:
Blemished skin

Tips: Pick dandelion leaves far away from roads and other polluted areas. Make sure they have not been sprayed with any pesticides — you don't want any undesirable substances in your oil.

This oil must be stored away from light to maintain its effectiveness. A cool, dark cupboard is the perfect place for the bottle between uses.

Note: Exact measurements are important when you're making skin- and hair-care products. Turn to page 17 for how-tos.

0.35 oz	fresh dandelion leaves (see tips, at left)	10 g
3.5 oz	argan oil	100 g

1. Wash dandelion leaves well and spin or pat dry. Using a sharp knife and a cutting board, chop dandelion leaves.

2. In a saucepan, heat argan oil over medium heat without letting oil start to smoke. Add chopped dandelion leaves and cook, stirring, for 10 minutes. Remove from heat. Let cool completely.

3. Using a fine-mesh sieve lined with cheesecloth, strain oil into a glass jar. Seal tightly. Store in a cool, dark place.

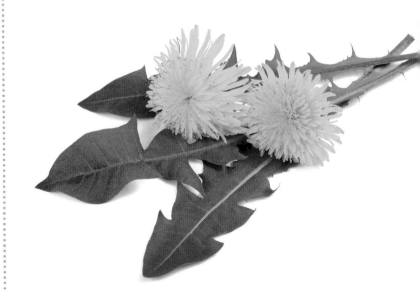

139

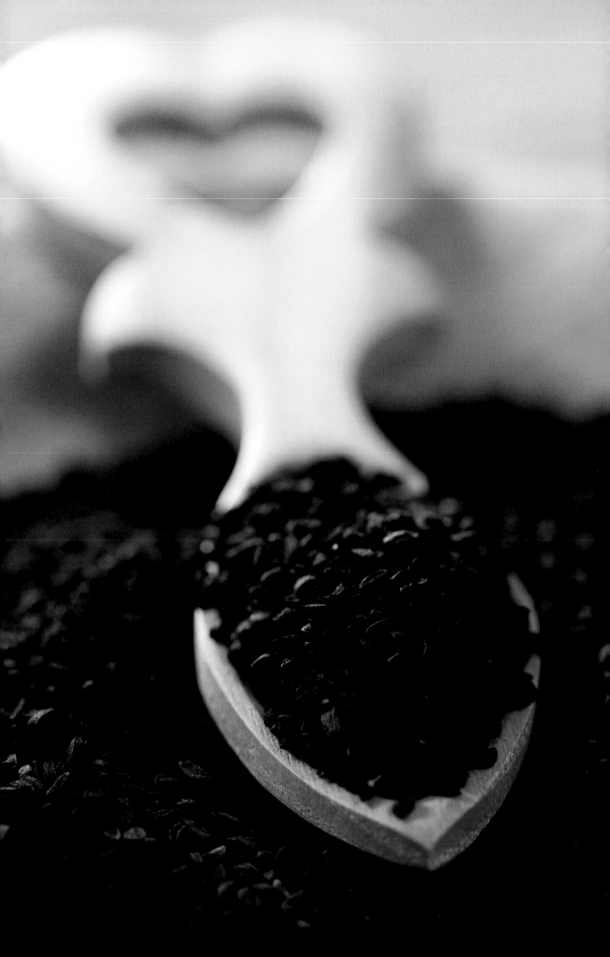

Black Cumin Oil

The therapeutic and cosmetic properties of the black cumin seed and its oil have been recognized since antiquity.

This health-enhancing oil is made from the seeds of the black cumin *(Nigella sativa)* plant. The plant has many common names, including black caraway flower, nutmeg flower, fennel flower and Roman coriander. The oil is known as black cumin oil or, simply, black seed oil.

The plant is native to Syria, but grows abundantly throughout the Mediterranean region. Today, it is cultivated from the Middle East to India, where it is widely used in Ayurvedic medicine. Black cumin seed was traditionally called "blessed seed" or "miracle seed." The ancient Egyptians are known to have used black cumin oil; it was found in Tutankhamen's tomb, and Cleopatra used it to enhance her beauty.

Black cumin oil is extracted from the seeds via cold pressing. It can be used alone or mixed with other oils. It is suitable for all skin types, even for people with skin problems. Black cumin oil is rich in vitamins A and E, beta-carotene, minerals and polyunsaturated fatty acids. It contains upwards of 100 components (many of which are unknown), including antibacterial and antiviral compounds.

Black cumin oil is beneficial in treating allergies and respiratory diseases, such as bronchitis, pharyngitis, laryngitis and asthma. It works as an expectorant to improve cold and flu symptoms. Black cumin oil is also used to treat rheumatic pain, migraines, back and joint pain, bruises and sprains. It fights fungal infections on the skin, and regular use can lighten the skin tone, if desired. Another bonus is that it's very good at improving acne and acts as a skin regenerator.

Black Cumin Pain-Relieving Oil

A combination of this warm oil and a gentle massage can soothe many types of pain. Rest and relax when you're done, to speed healing.

Best for: Back and joint pain, bruises and sprains

Note: Exact measurements are important when you're making skin- and hair-care products. Turn to page 17 for how-tos.

Caution: Do not use rosemary essential oil if you have epilepsy or high blood pressure.

1 oz	black cumin oil	30 g
5	drops rosemary essential oil (see caution, at left)	5
5	drops chamomile essential oil (see tip, below)	5
5	drops marjoram essential oil	5
5	drops thyme essential oil	5

1. In a saucepan, heat black cumin oil over low heat until warm without letting it start to smoke.

2. Using a wooden spoon, stir in rosemary, chamomile, marjoram and thyme essential oils. Use immediately.

Tip: You'll often find two types of chamomile essential oil at cosmetic-supply stores: German and Roman. They come from different strains of the chamomile plant, but both are soothing additions to homemade skin- and hair-care products.

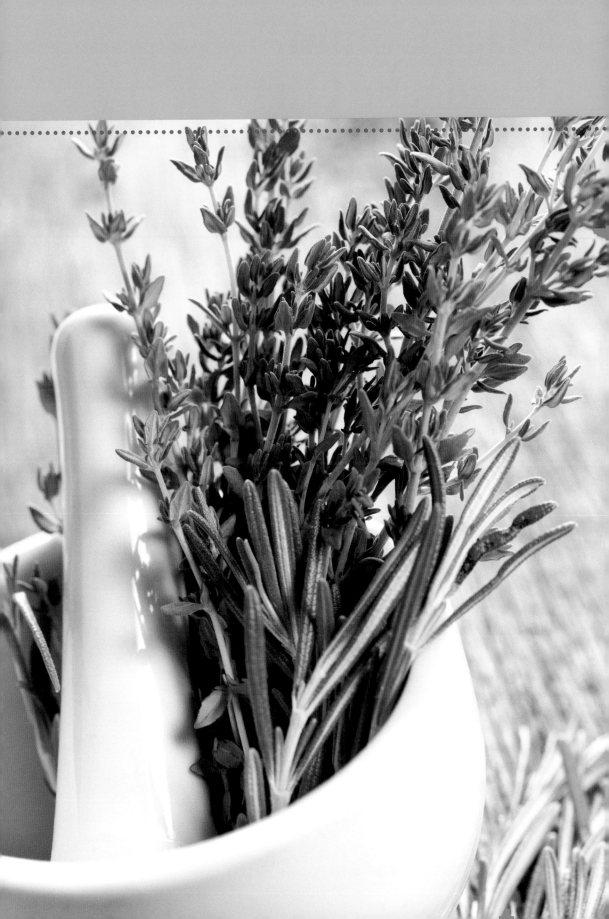

Black Cumin Headache Oil

When your head is pounding, you need relief quickly. This oil, combined with a soothing massage, can help.

Best for:
Headaches and migraine pain

0.35 oz	black cumin oil	10 g
5	drops lavender essential oil	5
2	drops clove essential oil	2

1. In a small bowl, combine black cumin oil, and lavender and clove essential oils.

2. Using a wooden spoon, stir until well combined. Use immediately.

Tip: Gently massage the oil over the affected area, such as the temples or neck.

Black Cumin Joint-Pain Oil

Rheumatic diseases and arthritis can wreak havoc on the joints. Gently massage this oil over trouble spots until it's completely absorbed, to help ease soreness.

Best for: Achy, sore joints

| 0.35 oz | black cumin oil | 10 g |
| 5 | drops ginger essential oil | 5 |

1. In a saucepan, heat black cumin oil over low heat until warm without letting it start to smoke.

2. Using a wooden spoon, stir in ginger essential oil. Use immediately.

Black Cumin Antifungal Skin Oil

Fungal infections on the skin can be very annoying. Massage this oil into the affected area daily, and the fungus will soon disappear.

Best for: Fungal infections on the skin

0.35 oz	black cumin oil	10 g
10	drops tea tree essential oil	10

1. Pour black cumin oil and tea tree essential oil into a small glass bottle. Seal tightly.

2. Shake to combine.

Black Cumin Acne-Fighting Oil

It might seem counterintuitive to use oil to treat acne, but this one works. Massage two or three drops into inflamed skin every night for amazing results.

Best for: Acne-prone skin

0.7 oz	black cumin oil	20 g
5	drops tea tree essential oil	5
5	drops citronella essential oil	5

1. Pour black cumin oil, and tea tree and citronella essential oils into a small glass bottle. Seal tightly.

2. Shake to combine.

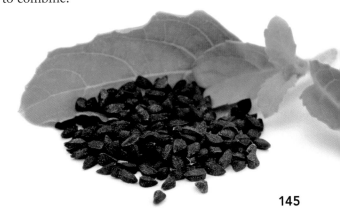

Black Cumin Soothing Eye Oil

This oil magically soothes sore, burning skin around the eyes that's caused by seasonal allergies, sties and minor irritations. Use your fingertips to spread the oil around your eye sockets, taking care not to get it in your eyes.

Best for: Sore, burning skin around the eyes

Note: Exact measurements are important when you're making skin- and hair-care products. Turn to page 17 for how-tos.

0.07 oz	black cumin oil	2 g
1	drop chamomile essential oil (see tip, below)	1

1. Combine black cumin oil and chamomile essential oil in a small bowl.
2. Stir until combined. Use immediately.

Tip: You'll often find two types of chamomile essential oil at cosmetic-supply stores: German and Roman. They come from different strains of the chamomile plant, but both are soothing additions to homemade skin- and hair-care products.

Lighten and Brighten Your Skin with Black Cumin Oil

Black cumin oil, used on its own, is wonderful at brightening and lightening facial skin. Moisten a cotton ball with the oil and wipe it gently over your face and neck, leaving it on for a minute or two. Rinse your face with plenty of cold water and gently pat dry to avoid blotting all the oil.

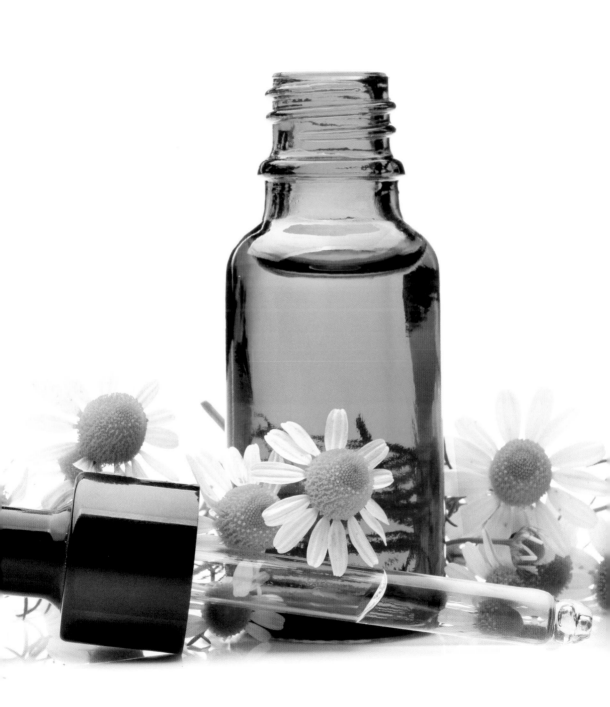

Black Cumin Soothing Ear Oil

Achy ears are so painful. This gentle oil helps relieve the pain and offers comfort while you're waiting to see the doctor.

Best for: Ear pain and inflammation

Note: Exact measurements are important when you're making skin- and hair-care products. Turn to page 17 for how-tos.

| 4 | drops black cumin oil | 4 |
| 4 | drops olive oil (see tips, below) | 4 |

1. In a small microwave-safe bowl, combine black cumin oil and olive oil.

2. Heat 1 second at a time just until slightly warmed. Use immediately.

Tips: Choose extra-virgin or virgin oils made from the first cold pressing.

To apply, place four drops in one ear and insert a small piece of cotton. Tilt your head to the opposite side for a few minutes to keep the oil in. Repeat with the other ear.

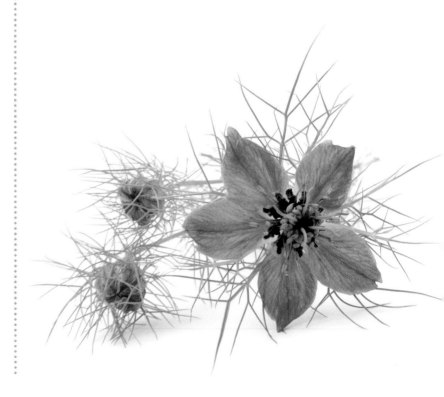

Black Cumin Inhalation Oil

Colds and flus can make you so stuffy and miserable. A steamy inhalation prepared with this oil will open up all those clogged areas and make breathing easier.

Best for: Colds and flus with head and/or chest congestion

Tip: The essential oils you use for skin- and hair-care products must be 100% pure. Don't use synthetic scents or oils, or essences designed for use in fragrance burners or lamp rings.

Note: Exact measurements are important when you're making skin- and hair-care products. Turn to page 17 for how-tos.

1 oz	black cumin oil	30 g
3	drops eucalyptus essential oil (see tip, at left)	3
3	drops tea tree essential oil	3
3	drops thyme essential oil	3
3	drops pine essential oil	3
3	drops peppermint essential oil	3

1. Pour black cumin oil, and eucalyptus, tea tree, thyme, pine and peppermint essential oils into a small glass bottle. Seal tightly.

2. Shake to combine.

3. In a large saucepan, bring 8 cups (2 L) water to a boil. Pour into a large wide-mouthed bowl and add a few drops of the oil mixture.

4. Drape a towel over your head and the bowl to enclose the fragrant steam. With your nostrils wide open, breathe slowly and deeply.

Tip: Use this inhalation treatment whenever you have bronchitis, a sore throat, a cough or congestion due to a cold or the flu. Another option is to rub a little bit of the oil mixture between your hands until warm and massage it into your neck and chest until it penetrates the skin. You can alternate between the two methods for an even more effective treatment.

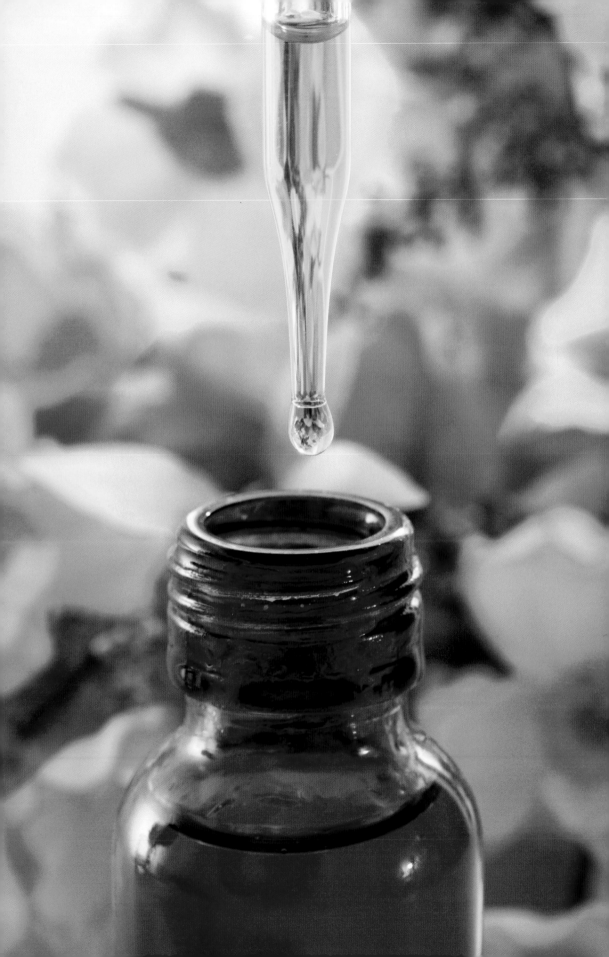

Andiroba Oil

Use andiroba oil to warm up the muscles and joints before playing sports or exercising on cold winter days.

The andiroba *(Carapa guianensis)* is a magnificent tree that grows in the Amazon rainforest. Andiroba oil, light amber in color, is cold pressed from the seeds.

The people of the Amazon region have used it for centuries, and they discovered its medicinal and cosmetic properties. They use this wonderful oil to protect their skin from cold, rain and insect bites that cause parasitic diseases. Indigenous women from the region also use the oil to massage areas plagued by fluid retention and cellulite.

Andiroba oil is very effective at repelling insects, including ticks and lice. The oil also has anti-inflammatory, antiseptic and antibacterial properties. It helps with wound healing and warms the skin and muscles, which keeps them from contracting and causing pain. Andiroba oil also makes hair soft and shiny. Its slippery texture makes it ideal for use in full-body massages, at home or at the spa.

Andiroba Healing Ointment

0.7 oz	green clay (see tip, below)	20 g
0.35 oz	andiroba oil	10 g
4	drops rosemary essential oil (see caution, below)	4

1. Combine green clay, andiroba oil and rosemary essential oil in a bowl.

2. Using a wooden spoon, stir well until ingredients are combined. Use immediately.

Tip: Green clay is often added to facial masks and treatments, and is thought to stimulate blood flow to injured areas and speed up the healing process. Look for it in powdered form at cosmetic-supply stores.

Caution: Do not use rosemary essential oil if you have epilepsy or high blood pressure.

Want to fix an injury fast? Apply this ointment, let it stand on the skin for about 15 minutes until it's completely dry, then wash off the mixture. Repeat daily until the injury is better.

Best for: Bruises, hematomas and swollen skin

Andiroba Hair Repair Oil

0.35 oz	andiroba oil	10 g
0.07 oz	pure vitamin E (see tip, below)	2 g

1. Pour andiroba oil and vitamin E into a small glass bottle. Seal tightly.

2. Shake well to combine.

Tip: Look for pure vitamin E in liquid form at cosmetic-supply stores. It's also easy to find online.

This oil heals hair that's been damaged by the intense heat of flat irons and blow dryers. Place a few drops of the oil on your fingertips and massage it through the hair before heat-styling, for silky results.

Best for: Dry and/or damaged hair

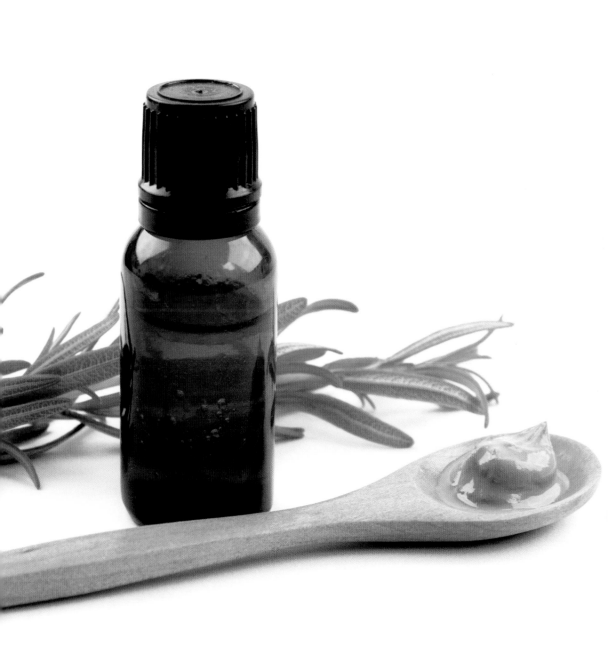

Andiroba Insect Repellent

If you're heading outside in the spring or summer, you'll surely be exposed to mosquitoes and other biting or stinging insects. Banish them by spreading this protective oil on your arms, legs and face.

Best for: All skin types

Tip: Store the finished oil away from light to keep its healing properties intact. This is a smart policy for all homemade oils.

Note: Exact measurements are important when you're making skin- and hair-care products. Turn to page 17 for how-tos.

| 0.7 oz | andiroba oil | 20 g |
| 0.04 oz | tea tree essential oil | 1 g |

1. Pour andiroba oil and tea tree essential oil into a small glass bottle. Seal tightly.
2. Shake to combine.

Andiroba Oil Keeps Lice Away

This oil can't treat a lice infestation once it has started, but it is excellent at preventing the bugs from taking up residence in the first place. Simply place a few drops of andiroba oil on your fingertips and distribute it evenly through your hair. Children heading to school are particularly susceptible, so treat them every morning before they leave home.

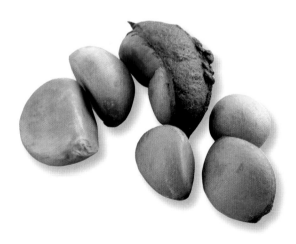

Andiroba Muscle Pain Oil

Massage is often the first line of treatment for sore muscles. Use a bit of this healing oil and massage the affected area two or three times a day for relief.

Best for: Cramped or sore muscles

1 oz	andiroba oil	30 g
5	drops rosemary essential oil (see caution, below)	5
5	drops cedar essential oil	5

1. Pour andiroba oil, and rosemary and cedar essential oils into a small glass bottle. Seal tightly.
2. Shake to combine.

Caution: Do not use rosemary essential oil if you have epilepsy or high blood pressure.

Andiroba Insect Bite Oil

Take the stinging and burning out of bug bites quickly. This oil-and-ammonia mix zaps the pain and itch immediately. Apply several times a day until discomfort passes.

Best for: Itchy, sore insect bites

| 0.18 oz | andiroba oil | 5 g |
| 2 | drops household ammonia (see tip, below) | 2 |

1. Pour andiroba oil and ammonia into a small glass bottle. Seal tightly.
2. Shake to combine.

Tip: You'll find bottles of household ammonia in the cleaning aisle of the supermarket. The fumes are incredibly strong, so hold the neck of the bottle away from your face as you open it.

Andiroba Anti-Cellulite Cream

This cream is excellent for treating cellulite and localized fluid retention, as well as areas with unsightly fat deposits. It also helps improve circulation. Apply once a day, massaging quickly and lightly until the cream is absorbed.

Best for: Cellulite-prone areas

Note: Exact measurements are important when you're making skin- and hair-care products. Turn to page 17 for how-tos.

1 oz	andiroba oil	30 g
0.4 oz	Lanette wax (see box, page 15)	12 g
12.3 oz	witch hazel	350 g
4	pinches citric acid powder (see box, page 27)	4
4	pinches ascorbic acid powder	4
12	drops geranium essential oil	12
10	drops fennel essential oil	10
10	drops grapefruit essential oil	10
10	drops cypress essential oil	10

1. Combine andiroba oil and Lanette wax in a saucepan. Heat over low heat just until ingredients are completely melted. Remove from heat and keep warm.

2. Pour witch hazel into a separate saucepan. Heat until lukewarm. Using a wooden spoon, stir in citric acid and ascorbic acid until dissolved.

3. Stir witch hazel mixture into oil mixture. Using a hand mixer, beat at low speed for 1 to 2 minutes. Let stand for 10 minutes.

4. Stir in geranium, fennel, grapefruit and cypress essential oils. Using a hand mixer, beat at high speed for 1 minute.

5. Pour or spoon mixture into glass jars. Let cool.

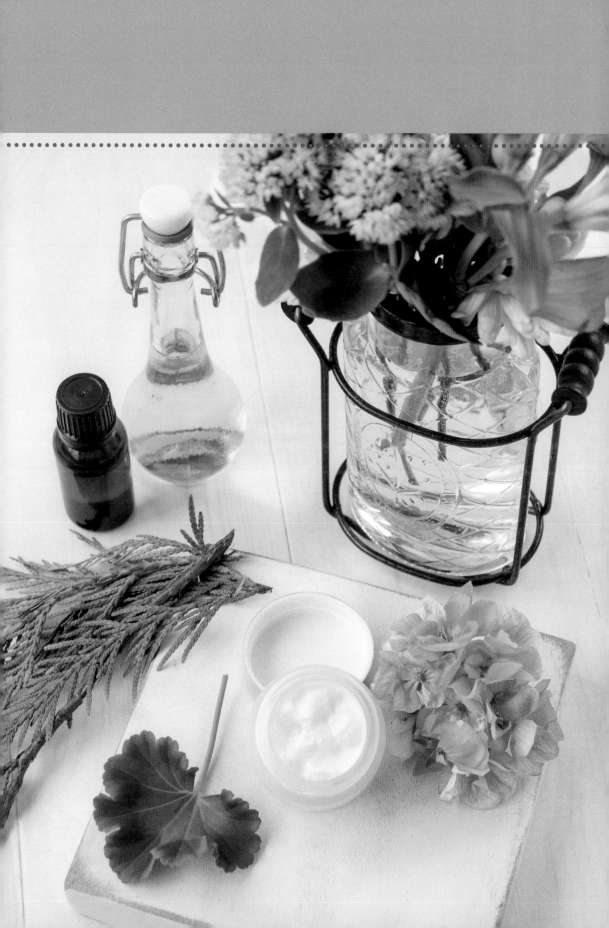

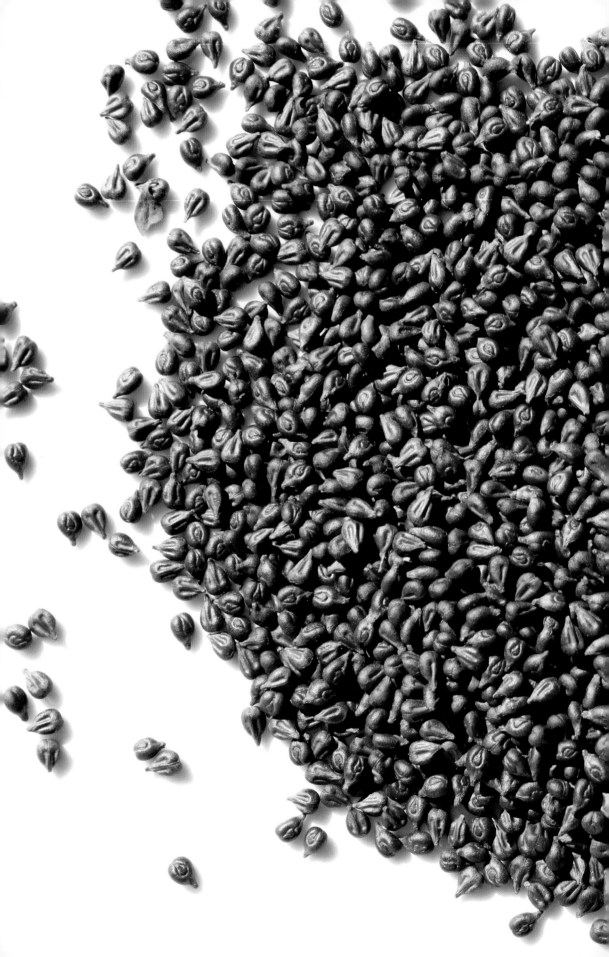

Grapeseed Oil

The main skin-care benefit of grapeseed oil is its significant antiaging powers.

The grapevine *(Vitis vinifera)* was one of the first plants cultivated by humans. In ancient Egypt, the custom of decorating temples with vine leaves was widespread. Many historians have pinpointed the grapevine's origin in the area around the Caspian Sea in Asia Minor, from which it spread throughout most of the other continents on the planet.

The fruit, leaves and branches of the grapevine have been employed since antiquity for medicinal uses. Today, there are holistic beauty treatments that call for grape skins, crushed seeds or even wine.

Grapeseed oil is, as its name implies, extracted from the seeds of grapes. It is dark green and strongly flavored, and it has a multitude of uses in the kitchen, showing up in everything from sauces to marinades. Grapeseed oil is good for frying because it has a high smoke point. But because it is one of the more expensive oils, it is also often used raw instead of in cooking, usually as a featured ingredient so that its flavor can be enjoyed.

Grapeseed oil contains essential fatty acids, including about 70% omega-6 linoleic acid and 18% omega-9 oleic acid, which, among many other benefits, help slow down skin aging. The oil is also high in vitamin E and bioflavonoids, powerful antioxidants that are excellent for skin health and counteract free radicals in the body. Grapeseed oil is recommended for all skin types, because it doesn't leave behind a greasy feeling and it is noncomedogenic (meaning it won't clog pores).

Grapeseed and Rose Hip Anti-Wrinkle Face Cream

Giving your skin the nutrients it needs to repair itself is so important. This cream is recommended for deep nutrition to banish wrinkles.

Best for: Dry or wrinkled skin

Tip: Liquid glycerin is a moisturizing ingredient often included in cosmetics, soaps, shampoos and creams. You'll find small bottles of it at drugstores, but cosmetic-supply stores sell larger bulk amounts.

Note: Exact measurements are important when you're making skin- and hair-care products. Turn to page 17 for how-tos.

0.7 oz	grapeseed oil	20 g
0.2 oz	Lanette wax (see box, page 15)	6 g
0.18 oz	cocoa butter	5 g
0.1 oz	jojoba oil	3 g
6 oz	mineral water	170 g
2	pinches citric acid powder (see box, page 27)	2
2	pinches ascorbic acid powder	2
0.18 oz	liquid glycerin (see tip, at left)	5 g
0.18 oz	rose hip seed oil	5 g
10	drops frankincense essential oil	10

1. Combine grapeseed oil, Lanette wax, cocoa butter and jojoba oil in a saucepan. Heat over low heat just until ingredients are completely melted. Remove from heat and keep warm.

2. Pour mineral water into a separate saucepan. Heat until lukewarm. Using a wooden spoon, stir in citric acid and ascorbic acid until dissolved.

3. Stir mineral water mixture into oil mixture. Using a hand mixer, beat at low speed for 1 to 2 minutes. Let stand for 10 minutes.

4. Stir in glycerin, rose hip seed oil and frankincense essential oil. Using a hand mixer, beat at high speed for 1 minute.

5. Pour or spoon mixture into glass jars. Let cool.

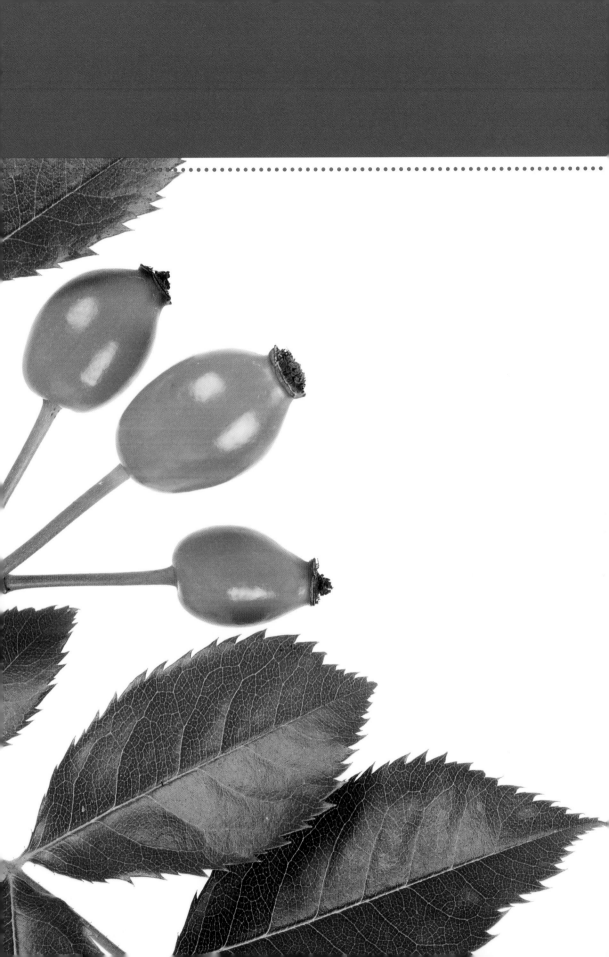

Grapeseed Moisturizing Anti-Wrinkle Face Cream

You can use this creamy potion to prevent wrinkles from starting, but it also does a nice job of reducing the appearance of ones that are already there.

Best for: Dry or wrinkled skin

Tip: Look for chunks or blocks of pure cocoa butter at cosmetic-supply stores. If you're using a large amount in a recipe, chop it up before adding it to the saucepan so it will melt more quickly.

Note: Exact measurements are important when you're making skin- and hair-care products. Turn to page 17 for how-tos.

0.7 oz	grapeseed oil	20 g
0.2 oz	Lanette wax (see box, page 15)	6 g
0.18 oz	cocoa butter (see tip, at left)	5 g
5.6 oz	rose water	160 g
2	pinches citric acid powder (see box, page 27)	2
2	pinches ascorbic acid powder	2
0.18 oz	liquid glycerin (see tips, below)	5 g
0.04 oz	pure vitamin A (see tips, below)	1 g
0.04 oz	pure vitamin E	1 g
7	drops geranium essential oil	7

1. Combine grapeseed oil, Lanette wax and cocoa butter in a saucepan. Heat over low heat just until ingredients are completely melted. Remove from heat and keep warm.

2. Pour rose water into a separate saucepan. Heat until lukewarm. Using a wooden spoon, stir in citric acid and ascorbic acid until dissolved.

3. Stir rose water mixture into oil mixture. Using a hand mixer, beat at low speed for 1 to 2 minutes. Let stand for 10 minutes.

4. Stir in glycerin, vitamins A and E, and geranium essential oil. Using a hand mixer, beat at high speed for 1 minute.

5. Pour or spoon mixture into glass jars. Let cool.

Tips: Liquid glycerin is a moisturizing ingredient often included in cosmetics, soaps, shampoos and creams. You'll find small bottles of it at drugstores, but cosmetic-supply stores sell larger bulk amounts.

Look for pure vitamins A and E in liquid form at cosmetic-supply stores. They're also easy to buy online.

Grapeseed Anti-Wrinkle Eye Cream

Use this rich cream to defend the delicate area around the eyes from the dreaded crow's-feet.

Best for: Wrinkles around the eyes

Tip: Rose water is often used in Middle Eastern and Mediterranean cooking. Look for it in Middle Eastern grocery stores and some well-stocked supermarkets.

Note: Exact measurements are important when you're making skin- and hair-care products. Turn to page 17 for how-tos.

0.35 oz	grapeseed oil	10 g
0.35 oz	sunflower oil	10 g
0.1 oz	Lanette wax (see box, page 15)	3 g
2.7 oz	rose water (see tip, at left)	77 g
1	pinch ascorbic acid powder (see box, page 27)	1
2	drops myrrh essential oil	2

1. Combine grapeseed oil, sunflower oil and Lanette wax in a saucepan. Heat over low heat just until ingredients are completely melted. Remove from heat and keep warm.

2. Pour rose water into a separate saucepan. Heat until lukewarm. Using a wooden spoon, stir in ascorbic acid until dissolved.

3. Stir rose water mixture into oil mixture. Using a hand mixer, beat at low speed for 1 to 2 minutes. Let stand for 10 minutes.

4. Stir in myrrh essential oil. Using a hand mixer, beat at high speed for 1 minute.

5. Pour or spoon mixture into glass jars. Let cool.

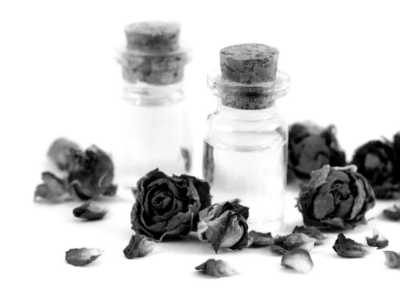

Grapeseed and Jojoba Moisturizing Acne Cream

Soothe acne and improve the appearance of skin by applying this cream every morning. Above all, be consistent in cleansing the skin of impurities before you moisturize.

Best for: Acne-prone skin

Tip: Store essential oils in a cool, dark place. Light exposure can diminish their healing properties.

Note: Exact measurements are important when you're making skin- and hair-care products. Turn to page 17 for how-tos.

0.2 oz	Lanette wax (see box, page 15)	6 g
0.18 oz	grapeseed oil	5 g
0.18 oz	jojoba oil	5 g
0.18 oz	cocoa butter	5 g
6.5 oz	mineral water	185 g
2	pinches citric acid powder (see box, page 27)	2
2	pinches ascorbic acid powder	2
6	drops cedar essential oil (see tip, at left)	6
6	drops bergamot essential oil	6

1. Combine Lanette wax, grapeseed oil, jojoba oil and cocoa butter in a saucepan. Heat over low heat just until ingredients are completely melted. Remove from heat and keep warm.

2. Pour mineral water into a separate saucepan. Heat until lukewarm. Using a wooden spoon, stir in citric acid and ascorbic acid until dissolved.

3. Stir mineral water mixture into oil mixture. Using a hand mixer, beat at low speed for 1 to 2 minutes. Let stand for 10 minutes.

4. Stir in cedar and bergamot essential oils. Using a hand mixer, beat at high speed for 1 minute.

5. Pour or spoon mixture into glass jars. Let cool.

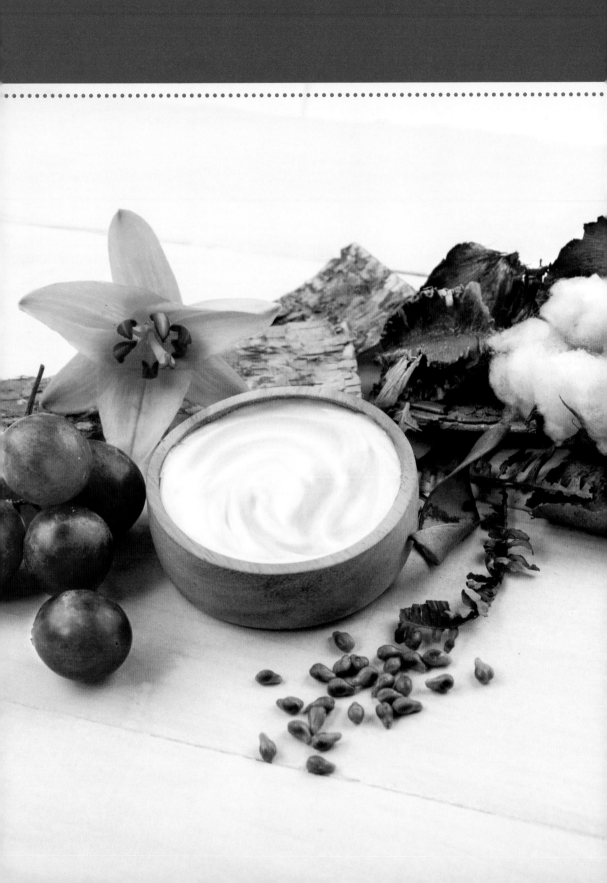

Grapeseed and Sesame Nourishing Acne Cream

Acne-prone skin needs good nutrition, like all skin. In general, apply nourishing creams about two hours before going to bed.

Best for: Acne-prone skin

Tip: Look for chunks or blocks of pure cocoa butter at cosmetic-supply stores. If you're using a large amount in a recipe, chop it up before adding it to the saucepan so it will melt more quickly.

Note: Exact measurements are important when you're making skin- and hair-care products. Turn to page 17 for how-tos.

0.2 oz	Lanette wax (see box, page 15)	6 g
0.18 oz	grapeseed oil	5 g
0.18 oz	sesame oil	5 g
0.18 oz	cocoa butter (see tip, at left)	5 g
6.3 oz	mineral water	180 g
2	pinches citric acid powder (see box, page 27)	2
2	pinches ascorbic acid powder	2
7	drops tea tree essential oil	7
6	drops cypress essential oil	6

1. Combine Lanette wax, grapeseed oil, sesame oil and cocoa butter in a saucepan. Heat over low heat just until ingredients are completely melted. Remove from heat and keep warm.

2. Pour mineral water into a separate saucepan. Heat until lukewarm. Using a wooden spoon, stir in citric acid and ascorbic acid until dissolved.

3. Stir mineral water mixture into oil mixture. Using a hand mixer, beat at low speed for 1 to 2 minutes. Let stand for 10 minutes.

4. Stir in tea tree and cypress essential oils. Using a hand mixer, beat at high speed for 1 minute.

5. Pour or spoon mixture into glass jars. Let cool.

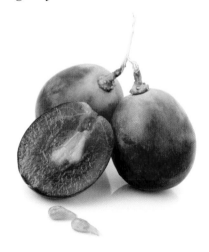

Grapeseed Anti-Wrinkle Body Cream

Everyone needs an easily absorbed, nourishing, restorative body cream. This one is the perfect choice to smooth on after a bath or shower.

Best for: Dry or wrinkled skin

Tip: Liquid glycerin is a moisturizing ingredient often included in cosmetics, soaps, shampoos and creams. You'll find small bottles of it at drugstores, but cosmetic-supply stores sell larger bulk amounts.

Note: Exact measurements are important when you're making skin- and hair-care products. Turn to page 17 for how-tos.

1 oz	grapeseed oil	30 g
0.4 oz	Lanette wax (see box, page 15)	12 g
0.35 oz	cocoa butter	10 g
12 oz	mineral water	340 g
4	pinches citric acid powder (see box, page 27)	4
4	pinches ascorbic acid powder	4
0.35 oz	liquid glycerin (see tip, at left)	10 g
15	drops cypress essential oil	15
15	drops lemongrass essential oil	15

1. Combine grapeseed oil, Lanette wax and cocoa butter in a saucepan. Heat over low heat just until ingredients are completely melted. Remove from heat and keep warm.

2. Pour mineral water into a separate saucepan. Heat until lukewarm. Using a wooden spoon, stir in citric acid and ascorbic acid until dissolved.

3. Stir mineral water mixture into oil mixture. Using a hand mixer, beat at low speed for 1 to 2 minutes. Let stand for 10 minutes.

4. Stir in glycerin, and cypress and lemongrass essential oils. Using a hand mixer, beat at high speed for 1 minute.

5. Pour or spoon mixture into glass jars. Let cool.

Grapeseed Stretch Mark–Reducing Oil

Stretch marks may not go away completely, but this oil will help them fade. Apply once a day, giving the area a gentle massage until the oil is absorbed.

Best for: Areas prone to stretch marks, such as the belly, thighs and buttocks

2.5 oz	grapeseed oil	70 g
1 oz	St. John's wort oil	30 g
0.7 oz	sesame oil	20 g
0.7 oz	rose hip seed oil	20 g
2	drops lemon essential oil	2

1. Pour grapeseed oil, St. John's wort oil, sesame oil, rose hip seed oil and lemon essential oil into a small glass bottle. Seal tightly.
2. Shake to combine.

Tip: Like most oils, this mixture is easier to apply if you pour it into a container with a roll-on top. It will dispense just the right amount.

Grapeseed Face and Body Scrub

Massage this scrub onto skin using a circular motion. Remove with warm water and soap, but don't wipe all the oil away. When you dry off, your skin will stay well moisturized.

Best for: All skin types

1 oz	cornmeal (see tip, below)	30 g
0.7 oz	grapeseed oil	20 g

1. Combine cornmeal and grapeseed oil in a bowl.
2. Using a wooden spoon, stir until ingredients are well combined. Use immediately.

Tip: Cornmeal is a terrific exfoliant. Choose a medium to coarse grind for best results in this scrub.

Grapeseed and Bergamot Makeup Remover

The citrusy scent of bergamot makes this simple makeup remover refreshing. Apply it as you would plain grapeseed oil (see box, at right).

Best for: All skin types

___

Note: Exact measurements are important when you're making skin- and hair-care products. Turn to page 17 for how-tos.

0.7 oz	grapeseed oil	20 g
3	drops bergamot essential oil	3

1. Pour grapeseed oil and bergamot essential oil into a small glass bottle. Seal tightly.

2. Shake to combine.

Grapeseed Oil Makes a Gentle Makeup Remover

You don't need to add anything to grapeseed oil to turn it into a good eye makeup remover. To apply it, dampen a cotton pad with a little water. Press it firmly between your palms to squeeze out the excess water. Add a little grapeseed oil to the cotton pad and lightly fold it to let the oil penetrate it thoroughly. Unfold and use the pad to wipe away makeup around the eyes.

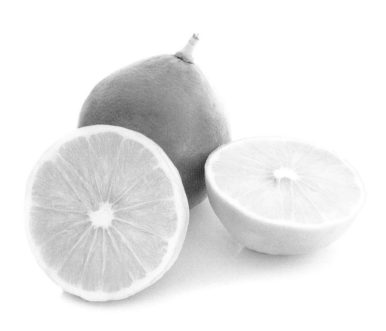

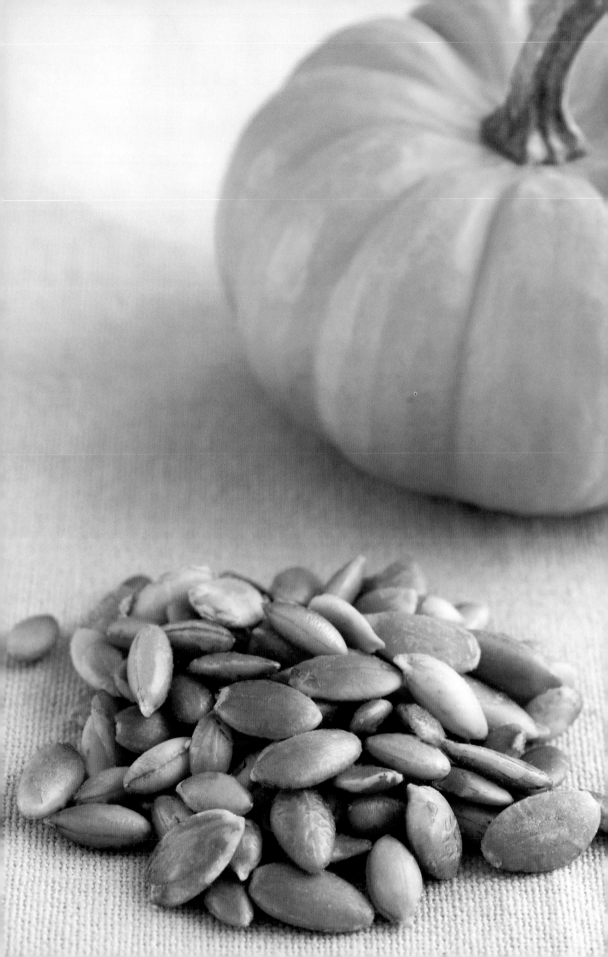

Pumpkin Seed Oil

Pumpkin seed oil is one of the well-known medicinal oils, and has been used in plant-based medicines for many years.

Pumpkin *(Cucurbita pepo)* belongs to the Cucurbitaceae family. Its seeds yield a splendid oil that can be used to cook gourmet dishes, but it's increasingly added to cosmetics for its countless skin-care benefits.

Pumpkin seed oil contains nearly 80% unsaturated fatty acids, especially omega-6 linoleic acid. It is rich in vitamins, particularly vitamins E and K, and minerals, including calcium, phosphorus, iron, potassium and zinc (which helps strengthen the immune system). Pumpkin seed oil also contains phytosterols and carotenes, so it is recommended for treating urinary tract problems. Pumpkin seeds have long been recommended for prostate problems, as well. And while this oil is rich in the well-known alpha-tocopherol, a type of vitamin E, it is even richer in delta-tocopherol, another form that is one of the most potent antioxidants.

In skin-care products, pumpkin seed oil is versatile and can be used in a wide variety of formulas. It is absorbed well and leaves no greasy feeling on the skin. It helps repair skin damage by protecting tissues from moisture loss and leaves them nourished and elastic.

Pumpkin Seed Moisturizing Face Cream

This cream is recommended for people of all ages with normal or combination skin. The orange essential oil gives it a fruity zing you'll enjoy in the morning.

Best for: Normal or combination skin

Tip: Liquid glycerin is a moisturizing ingredient often included in cosmetics, soaps, shampoos and creams. You'll find small bottles of it at drugstores, but cosmetic-supply stores sell larger bulk amounts.

Note: Exact measurements are important when you're making skin- and hair-care products. Turn to page 17 for how-tos.

0.7 oz	pumpkin seed oil	20 g
0.2 oz	Lanette wax (see box, page 15)	6 g
0.18 oz	cocoa butter	5 g
5.8 oz	rose water	165 g
2	pinches citric acid powder (see box, page 27)	2
2	pinches ascorbic acid powder	2
0.2 oz	liquid glycerin (see tip, at left)	6 g
10	drops orange essential oil	10

1. Combine pumpkin seed oil, Lanette wax and cocoa butter in a saucepan. Heat over low heat just until ingredients are completely melted. Remove from heat and keep warm.

2. Pour rose water into a separate saucepan. Heat until lukewarm. Using a wooden spoon, stir in citric acid and ascorbic acid until dissolved.

3. Stir rose water mixture into oil mixture. Using a hand mixer, beat at low speed for 1 to 2 minutes. Let stand for 10 minutes.

4. Stir in glycerin and orange essential oil. Using a hand mixer, beat at high speed for 1 minute.

5. Pour or spoon mixture into glass jars. Let cool.

Make Your Own Tinted Moisturizer

This cream is an excellent base for a tinted moisturizer, and you won't need foundation on top of it. Here's how to make it: measure 0.5 oz (15 g) Pumpkin Seed Moisturizing Face Cream (recipe, above) into a small bowl. Add about 0.04 oz (1 g) of your favorite tinted loose powder (adjust if necessary to reach the desired shade). Add 2 drops geranium essential oil and beat well to blend. It's that simple and made to order for your skin.

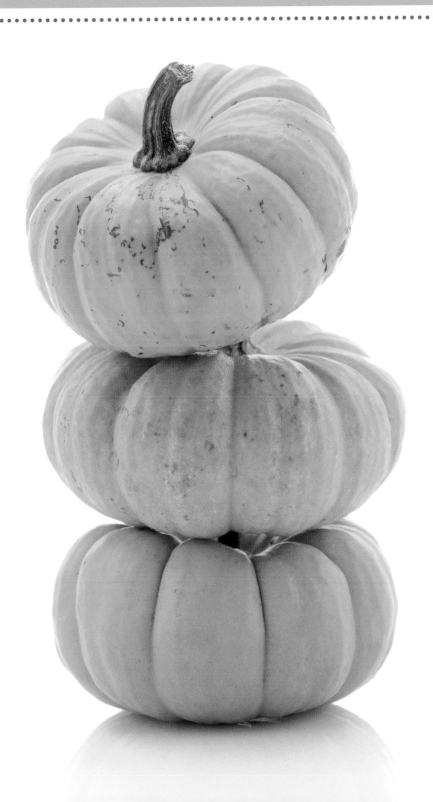

Pumpkin Seed Nourishing Face Cream

Like all nourishing creams, this should be applied two hours before retiring at night. You'll wake up feeling refreshed and beautiful.

Best for: Normal or combination skin

Note: Exact measurements are important when you're making skin- and hair-care products. Turn to page 17 for how-tos.

0.9 oz	pumpkin seed oil	25 g
0.2 oz	Lanette wax (see box, page 15)	6 g
0.18 oz	hazelnut oil	5 g
0.18 oz	cocoa butter	5 g
5.6 oz	mineral water	160 g
2	pinches citric acid powder (see box, page 27)	2
2	pinches ascorbic acid powder	2
15	drops frankincense essential oil	15

1. Combine pumpkin seed oil, Lanette wax, hazelnut oil and cocoa butter in a saucepan. Heat over low heat just until ingredients are completely melted. Remove from heat and keep warm.

2. Pour mineral water into a separate saucepan. Heat until lukewarm. Using a wooden spoon, stir in citric acid and ascorbic acid until dissolved.

3. Stir mineral water mixture into oil mixture. Using a hand mixer, beat at low speed for 1 to 2 minutes. Let stand for 10 minutes.

4. Stir in frankincense essential oil. Using a hand mixer, beat at high speed for 1 minute.

5. Pour or spoon mixture into glass jars. Let cool.

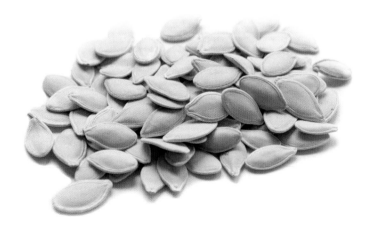

Pumpkin Seed Quick-Absorbing Hand Cream

An easily absorbed hand cream is best for daytime. This smooth formula won't leave your hands greasy, so you can go right back to work after applying it.

Best for: Dry hands

Tip: Citronella essential oil has a strong lemongrass-like aroma. It's often used in perfumes, and is a natural insect repellent.

Note: Exact measurements are important when you're making skin- and hair-care products. Turn to page 17 for how-tos.

0.35 oz	pumpkin seed oil	10 g
0.2 oz	Lanette wax (see box, page 15)	6 g
0.18 oz	cocoa butter	5 g
6 oz	witch hazel	170 g
2	pinches citric acid powder (see box, page 27)	2
2	pinches ascorbic acid powder	2
0.35 oz	liquid glycerin	10 g
15	drops citronella essential oil (see tip, at left)	15

1. Combine pumpkin seed oil, Lanette wax and cocoa butter in a saucepan. Heat over low heat just until ingredients are completely melted. Remove from heat and keep warm.

2. Pour witch hazel into a separate saucepan. Heat until lukewarm. Using a wooden spoon, stir in citric acid and ascorbic acid until dissolved.

3. Stir witch hazel mixture into oil mixture. Using a hand mixer, beat at low speed for 1 to 2 minutes. Let stand for 10 minutes.

4. Stir in glycerin and citronella essential oil. Using a hand mixer, beat at high speed for 1 minute.

5. Pour or spoon mixture into glass jars. Let cool.

Pumpkin Seed Bust Cream

This cream smooths your décolletage, and it can help prevent sagging from starting. As the saying goes, "An ounce of prevention is worth a pound of cure." To apply, spread cream gently over the bust area until completely absorbed. Use daily.

Best for: Sagging chest skin

Tip: There are many kinds of sage. Clary sage (*Salvia sclarea*) is one of the most commonly used varieties in skin-care formulas, and it has a wonderful flowery scent.

Note: Exact measurements are important when you're making skin- and hair-care products. Turn to page 17 for how-tos.

1.2 oz	pumpkin seed oil (see tip, below)	35 g
0.35 oz	cocoa butter	10 g
0.2 oz	Lanette wax (see box, page 15)	6 g
5.1 oz	witch hazel	145 g
2	pinches citric acid powder (see box, page 27)	2
2	pinches ascorbic acid powder	2
0.07 oz	pure vitamin A	2 g
7	drops clary sage essential oil (see tip, at left)	7
7	drops patchouli essential oil	7
7	drops lemon essential oil	7
7	drops lemongrass essential oil	7
7	drops rosewood essential oil (see tip, page 36)	7

1. Combine pumpkin seed oil, cocoa butter and Lanette wax in a saucepan. Heat over low heat just until ingredients are completely melted. Remove from heat and keep warm.

2. Pour witch hazel into a separate saucepan. Heat until lukewarm. Using a wooden spoon, stir in citric acid and ascorbic acid until dissolved.

3. Stir witch hazel mixture into oil mixture. Using a hand mixer, beat at low speed for 1 to 2 minutes. Let stand for 10 minutes.

4. Stir in vitamin A, and clary sage, patchouli, lemon, lemongrass and rosewood essential oils. Using a hand mixer, beat at high speed for 1 minute.

5. Pour or spoon mixture into glass jars. Let cool.

Tip: Pumpkin seed oil (sometimes called "green gold") gives this cream its brilliant green color. In the bottle, the oil appears very dark with hints of red. But if you see a thin layer of the oil (or see it when it has been mixed with pale ingredients), the deep green hue is visible.

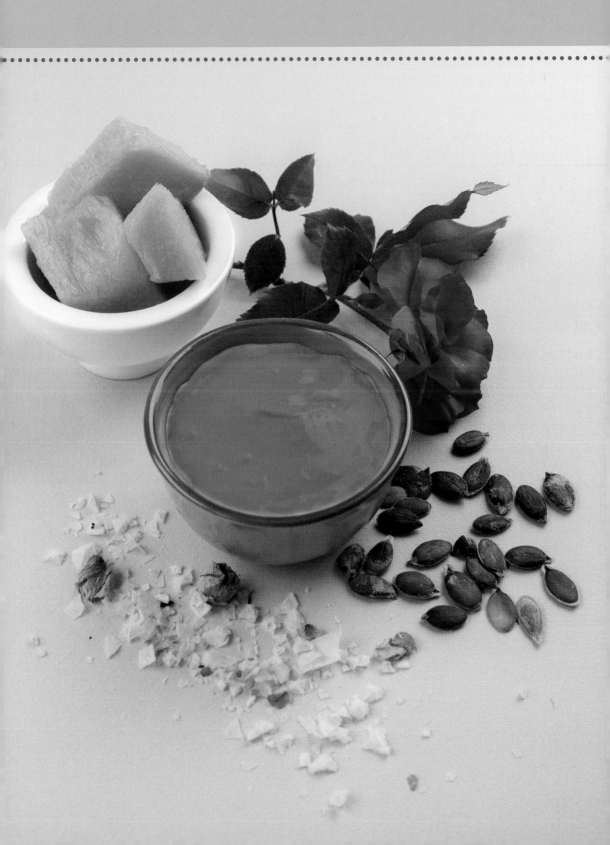

Pumpkin Seed and Grapefruit Body Cream

Smooth on this cream regularly, and you'll find it leaves your skin utterly soft and well moisturized.

Best for: Normal or combination skin

Tips: Orange flower water is also called orange blossom water. It's easy to find in Middle Eastern grocery stores and some well-stocked supermarkets, where it's sold for use in cooking.

Store essential oils in a cool, dark place to preserve their healing compounds. Light exposure weakens them.

Note: Exact measurements are important when you're making skin- and hair-care products. Turn to page 17 for how-tos.

0.7 oz	pumpkin seed oil	20 g
0.4 oz	Lanette wax (see box, page 15)	12 g
0.35 oz	cocoa butter	10 g
12.3 oz	orange flower water (see tips, at left)	350 g
4	pinches citric acid powder (see box, page 27)	4
4	pinches ascorbic acid powder	4
0.35 oz	liquid glycerin	10 g
20	drops grapefruit essential oil (see tips, at left)	20

1. Combine pumpkin seed oil, Lanette wax and cocoa butter in a saucepan. Heat over low heat just until ingredients are completely melted. Remove from heat and keep warm.

2. Pour orange flower water into a separate saucepan. Heat until lukewarm. Using a wooden spoon, stir in citric acid and ascorbic acid until dissolved.

3. Stir orange flower water mixture into oil mixture. Using a hand mixer, beat at low speed for 1 to 2 minutes. Let stand for 10 minutes.

4. Stir in glycerin and grapefruit essential oil. Using a hand mixer, beat at high speed for 1 minute.

5. Pour or spoon mixture into glass jars. Let cool.

Pumpkin Seed Stretch Mark–Fighting Cream

This cream works best on recent stretch marks created by pregnancy, weight loss and so on. Older stretch marks are more difficult to remove, but if you treat them daily with this cream, you will see noticeable improvement.

Best for: Areas prone to stretch marks, such as the belly, thighs and buttocks

Tip: Wheat germ oil is highly perishable. Store it in the refrigerator to keep it from going rancid.

Note: Exact measurements are important when you're making skin- and hair-care products. Turn to page 17 for how-tos.

0.35 oz	pumpkin seed oil	10 g
0.35 oz	wheat germ oil (see tip, at left)	10 g
0.2 oz	Lanette wax (see box, page 15)	6 g
0.1 oz	beeswax (see tips, below)	3 g
0.1 oz	lanolin (see tips, below)	3 g
5.6 oz	mineral water	160 g
2	pinches citric acid powder (see box, page 27)	2
2	pinches ascorbic acid powder	2
0.35 oz	rose hip seed oil	10 g
20	drops cedar essential oil	20

1. Combine pumpkin seed oil, wheat germ oil, Lanette wax, beeswax and lanolin in a saucepan. Heat over low heat just until ingredients are completely melted. Remove from heat and keep warm.

2. Pour mineral water into a separate saucepan. Heat until lukewarm. Using a wooden spoon, stir in citric acid and ascorbic acid until dissolved.

3. Stir mineral water mixture into oil mixture. Using a hand mixer, beat at low speed for 1 to 2 minutes. Let stand for 10 minutes.

4. Stir in rose hip seed oil and cedar essential oil. Using a hand mixer, beat at high speed for 1 minute.

5. Pour or spoon mixture into glass jars. Let cool.

Tips: Look for 100% pure beeswax that has been minimally processed. It is often sold in bulk, in chunks; if the recipe calls for a large amount, grate the wax so it will melt quickly and smoothly. Alternatively, you can buy beeswax that has been formed into pearls, which are easy to measure and melt quickly.

Lanolin is a waxy natural moisturizer derived from sheep's wool. It has long been used as a softening and moisturizing agent, especially in hand creams. You can find jars of it at cosmetic-supply stores. It has a distinctive, earthy aroma, and a little goes a long way.

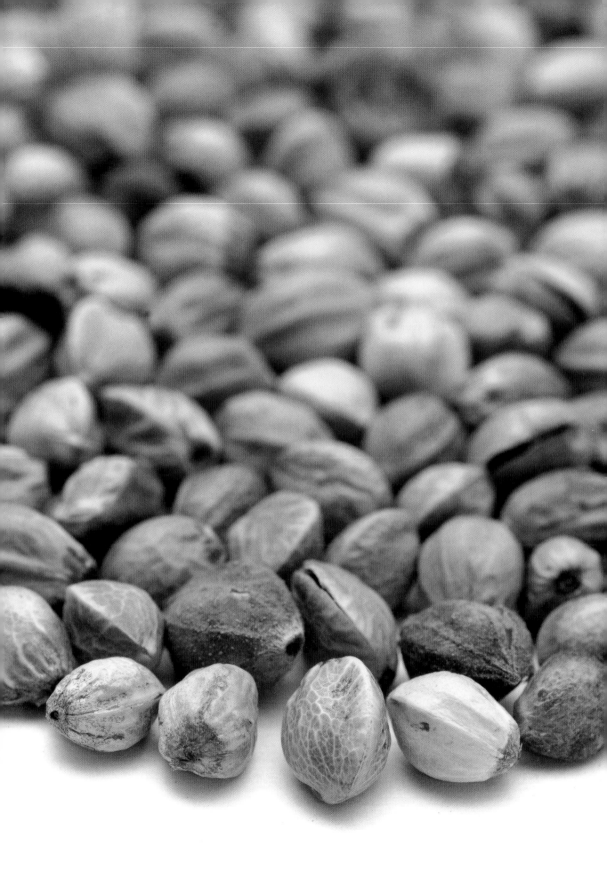

Hemp Seed Oil

Hemp seed oil offers so many benefits, for use in both food and body-care products. It seems to be approaching its heyday.

Hemp seed oil has been in use for more than 5,000 years. Hemp is thought to have been one of the first crops cultivated by humans. In ancient China, people used hemp seeds and their oil to treat skin inflammations. The oil is obtained by pressing the seeds of specific varieties of *Cannabis sativa*. The seeds of these varieties do not contain psychoactive substances, unlike the flowers and leaves of other strains of *Cannabis sativa* and *Cannabis indica*.

In the kitchen, hemp seed oil's nutty flavor lends itself to use in sauces, dressings and salads. Also, it is easily digested. The ratio of omega-6 to omega-3 fatty acids is the most balanced of all the oils: three parts omega-6 to one part omega-3. According to recent research, these are the best proportions for these fatty acids in food sources. In the typical Western diet, the ratio is usually closer to 10 to one, which is especially dangerous for cardiovascular health. Therefore, we should increase our consumption of omega-3 fatty acids — and hemp seed oil can be a part of that change.

In skin- and hair-care products, the oil is very popular because it produces significant improvements in sensitive and atopic (hypersensitive or allergy-prone) skin, especially in children. Hemp seed oil is also good for people with psoriasis or dermatitis.

With more and more studies coming out about its beneficial applications in both food and cosmetics, hemp seed oil has a promising future. It is heading for a boom, just like aloe vera had in its day.

Hemp Seed Moisturizing Face Cream

If your skin gets dried out the minute the temperature changes, this face cream is perfect for you. It's ideal on delicate skin, especially in kids.

Best for:
Sensitive or atopic (hypersensitive or allergy-prone) skin, and children's skin

Tip: Rose water is often used in Middle Eastern and Mediterranean cooking. Look for it in Middle Eastern grocery stores and some well-stocked supermarkets.

Note: Exact measurements are important when you're making skin- and hair-care products. Turn to page 17 for how-tos.

0.5 oz	hemp seed oil	15 g
0.35 oz	cocoa butter	10 g
0.2 oz	Lanette wax (see box, page 15)	6 g
5.8 oz	rose water (see tip, at left)	165 g
2	pinches citric acid powder (see box, page 27)	2
2	pinches ascorbic acid powder	2
0.28 oz	liquid glycerin	8 g
6	drops lavender essential oil	6

1. Combine hemp seed oil, cocoa butter and Lanette wax in a saucepan. Heat over low heat just until ingredients are completely melted. Remove from heat and keep warm.

2. Pour rose water into a separate saucepan. Heat until lukewarm. Using a wooden spoon, stir in citric acid and ascorbic acid until dissolved.

3. Stir rose water mixture into oil mixture. Using a hand mixer, beat at low speed for 1 to 2 minutes. Let stand for 10 minutes.

4. Stir in glycerin and lavender essential oil. Using a hand mixer, beat at high speed for 1 minute.

5. Pour or spoon mixture into glass jars. Let cool.

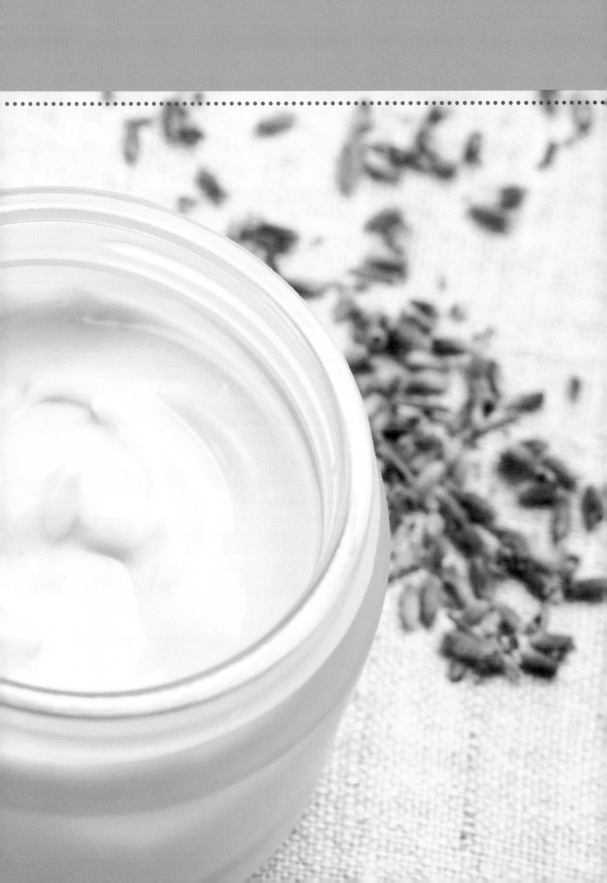

Hemp Seed Nourishing Face Cream

Skin that is sensitive, atopic or youthful needs deep nourishment, because it tends to lose moisture more quickly than other skin types.

Best for:
Sensitive or atopic (hypersensitive or allergy-prone) skin, and children's skin

Tips: Pure shea butter comes in chunks, like cocoa butter, at cosmetic-supply stores. Break or chop it up before adding it to the saucepan so that it melts quickly and easily.

Look for pure vitamin E in liquid form at cosmetic-supply stores. It's also easy to buy online.

Note: Exact measurements are important when you're making skin- and hair-care products. Turn to page 17 for how-tos.

0.7 oz	hemp seed oil	20 g
0.2 oz	Lanette wax (see box, page 15)	6 g
0.18 oz	shea butter (see tips, at left)	5 g
0.1 oz	wheat germ oil (see tip, page 179)	3 g
5.8 oz	mineral water	165 g
2	pinches citric acid powder (see box, page 27)	2
2	pinches ascorbic acid powder	2
0.1 oz	pure vitamin E (see tips, at left)	3 g
6	drops Roman chamomile essential oil	6

1. Combine hemp seed oil, Lanette wax, shea butter and wheat germ oil in a saucepan. Heat over low heat just until ingredients are completely melted. Remove from heat and keep warm.

2. Pour mineral water into a separate saucepan. Heat until lukewarm. Using a wooden spoon, stir in citric acid and ascorbic acid until dissolved.

3. Stir mineral water mixture into oil mixture. Using a hand mixer, beat at low speed for 1 to 2 minutes. Let stand for 10 minutes.

4. Stir in vitamin E and Roman chamomile essential oil. Using a hand mixer, beat at high speed for 1 minute.

5. Pour or spoon mixture into glass jars. Let cool.

Hemp Seed and Lavender Body Cream

You treat your face to moisturizer. Now make sure you treat your body to it, too, so any dryness is banished for good.

Best for:
Sensitive or atopic (hypersensitive or allergy-prone) skin, and children's skin

Note: Exact measurements are important when you're making skin- and hair-care products. Turn to page 17 for how-tos.

0.7 oz	hemp seed oil	20 g
0.5 oz	cocoa butter	15 g
0.4 oz	Lanette wax (see box, page 15)	12 g
0.18 oz	sweet almond oil	5 g
12.3 oz	mineral water	350 g
4	pinches citric acid powder (see box, page 27)	4
4	pinches ascorbic acid powder	4
10	drops lavender essential oil	10

1. Combine hemp seed oil, cocoa butter, Lanette wax and sweet almond oil in a saucepan. Heat over low heat just until ingredients are completely melted. Remove from heat and keep warm.

2. Pour mineral water into a separate saucepan. Heat until lukewarm. Using a wooden spoon, stir in citric acid and ascorbic acid until dissolved.

3. Stir mineral water mixture into oil mixture. Using a hand mixer, beat at low speed for 1 to 2 minutes. Let stand for 10 minutes.

4. Stir in lavender essential oil. Using a hand mixer, beat at high speed for 1 minute.

5. Pour or spoon mixture into glass jars. Let cool.

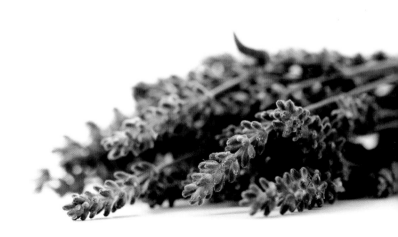

Hemp Seed and Rose Hip Shampoo

Fresh, fragrant and supremely gentle, this shampoo is good for even the most delicate scalps.

Best for:
Sensitive scalps and children's hair

Tip: Coco betaine (short for cocamido-propyl betaine) is a surfactant made from coconut oil and gives shampoos their cleaning power and lather. It's easy to find at cosmetic-supply stores.

Note: Exact measurements are important when you're making skin- and hair-care products. Turn to page 17 for how-tos.

2 to 3 tbsp	fresh rose hips (see tip, below)	30 to 45 mL
4.9 oz	mineral water	140 g
4.6 oz	coco betaine (see tip, at left)	130 g
0.1 oz	hemp seed oil	3 g
15	drops grapefruit essential oil	15

1. Place rose hips in a heatproof bowl. In a saucepan, bring mineral water to a boil. Pour boiling mineral water over rose hips. Cover and let steep for 10 minutes.

2. Using a fine-mesh sieve lined with cheesecloth, strain the rose hip infusion into a clean bowl. Let cool completely.

3. Pour infusion, coco betaine, hemp seed oil and grapefruit essential oil into a bottle. Seal tightly. Shake to combine.

Tip: Rose hips are the oval fruits created when a rose bush has finished flowering. Pick them from rose bushes that have not been sprayed with pesticides, or buy organic rose hips if you can find them.

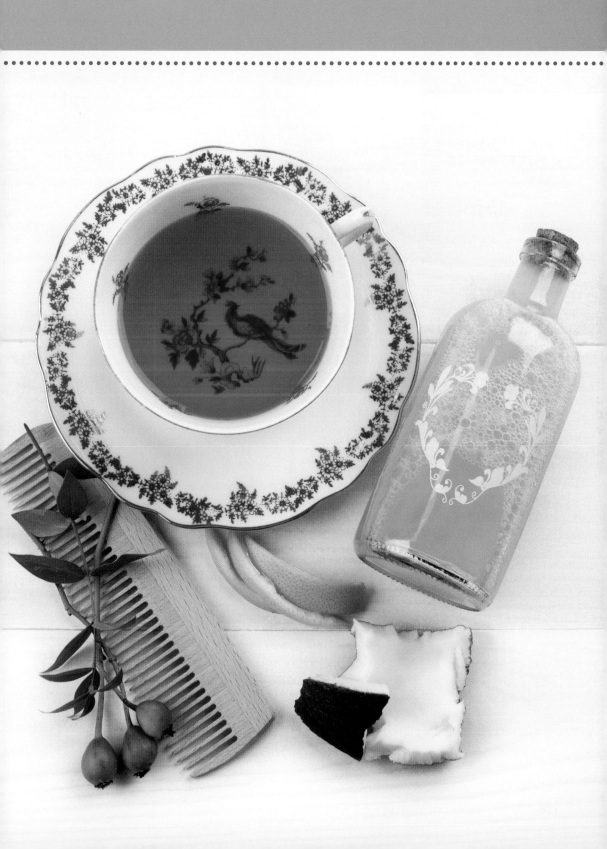

Hemp Seed and Sugar Exfoliating Scrub

Delicate, sensitive skin needs to be treated with care. Apply this scrub all over your body and face, then massage gently to moisturize and exfoliate at the same time.

Best for:
Sensitive or atopic (hypersensitive or allergy-prone) skin, and children's skin

2.5 oz	granulated sugar	70 g
1 oz	hemp seed oil	30 g
5	drops grapefruit essential oil	5

1. Combine sugar, hemp seed oil and grapefruit essential oil in a bowl.

2. Using a wooden spoon, stir until ingredients are well combined. Use immediately.

Hemp Seed Congestion-Fighting Oil

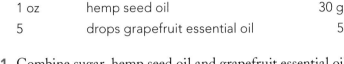

Colds, coughs and flus can all cause uncomfortable congestion. This treatment contains hemp seed oil plus two essential oils to help unclog your airways.

Best for: Colds and flus, with head and/or chest congestion

0.35 oz	hemp seed oil	10 g
12	drops frankincense essential oil	12
12	drops myrrh essential oil	12

1. Pour hemp seed oil, and frankincense and myrrh essential oils into a small glass bottle. Seal tightly.

2. Shake to combine. Rub a small amount over chest until completely absorbed.

Tip: Another way to use this oil is to inhale the vapor. In a large saucepan, bring 8 cups (2 L) water to a boil. Pour into a large wide-mouthed bowl and add a few drops of the oil mixture. Drape a towel over your head and the bowl to enclose the fragrant steam. With your nostrils wide open, breathe slowly and deeply.

Hemp Seed and Tea Tree Oil Hair Mask

For dry tresses, soak a cotton ball with this mixture and apply from roots to ends. For dermatitis, apply only to the scalp. Wrap your hair up in a towel and let stand for two hours, then wash as usual.

Best for: Dry to very dry hair, and flaky or dermatitis-prone scalps

| 1 oz | hemp seed oil | 30 g |
| 10 | drops tea tree essential oil | 10 |

1. Pour hemp seed oil and tea tree essential oil into a small glass bottle. Seal tightly.

2. Shake to combine.

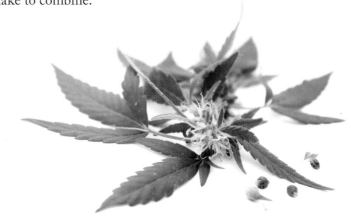

Hemp Seed Body Oil

Fresh-smelling and gentle, this oil calms irritations. It's excellent for anyone with delicate skin — especially kids.

Best for: Sensitive or atopic (hypersensitive or allergy-prone) skin, and children's skin

3.5 oz	hemp seed oil	100 g
10	drops Roman chamomile essential oil	10
5	drops lavandin essential oil (see tip, below)	5

1. Pour hemp seed oil, and Roman chamomile and lavandin essential oils into a small glass bottle. Seal tightly.

2. Shake to combine.

Tip: Lavandin (*Lavandula* x *intermedia*) is a hybrid of true lavender and spike lavender. It has different health-enhancing properties than regular lavender, and it's terrific for treating skin irritations.

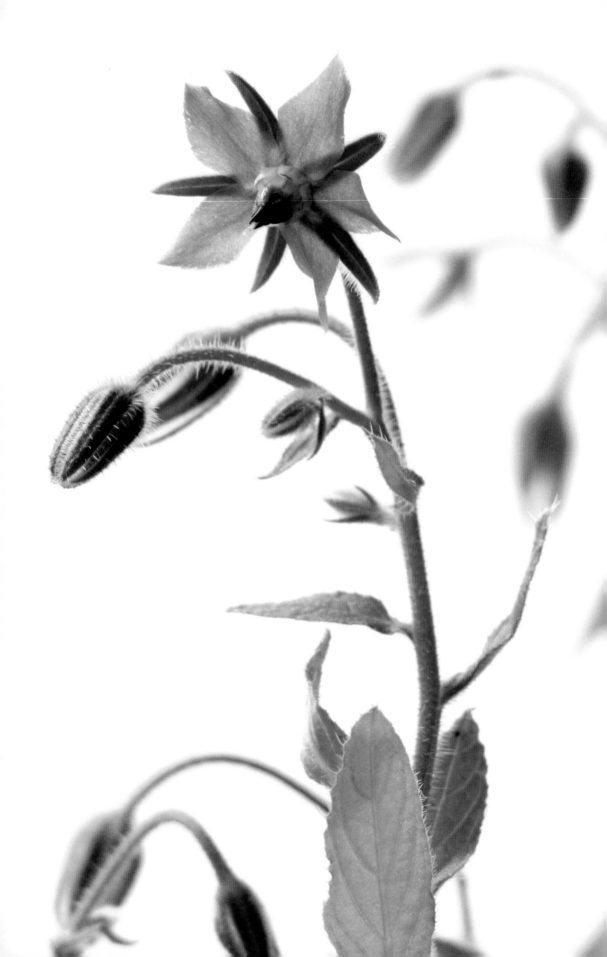

Borage Oil

Borage oil used topically smooths skin and helps prevent the formation of wrinkles. It can also repair damaged hair.

Borage *(Borago officinalis)* is a plant native to the Mediterranean region. Its beautiful blue, star-shaped flowers give it one of its common names, starflower.

The oil extracted from its seeds is rich in omega-6 fatty acids, especially gamma-linolenic acid and linoleic acid. Borage oil is often used in natural remedies because it has protective properties and an anti-inflammatory effect. It also offers notable skin- and hair-care benefits. Its action is most effective if taken in two ways: orally, to fight skin dryness from the inside, and externally (in an appropriate formula), to nourish problem skin from the outside.

Borage oil (sometimes labeled borage seed oil) is usually available in soft gel capsules in the supplement aisle of pharmacies, but you can get bottles of it from some cosmetic-supply or specialty oil stores online. To use the oil in the gel capsules, pierce them with a large, sharp sewing needle and squeeze out the contents. The highest-quality borage oil is obtained from the first cold pressing, like all extra-virgin or virgin oils. When extracted this way, the oil retains all of its beneficial properties.

Borage and Mallow Shampoo

A moisturizing shampoo like this is always good to have in your beauty toolkit. It gives dry hair a lovely sheen and smoothness.

Best for: Dry hair

Tips: Common mallow (*Malva sylvestris*) can be hard to find in the wild, but it grows well in pots at home if you want to use fresh flowers. Herbalists' shops often carry the dried version, which is more convenient.

Coco betaine (short for cocamidopropyl betaine) is a surfactant made from coconut oil and gives shampoos their cleaning power and lather. It's easy to find at cosmetic-supply stores.

Note: Exact measurements are important when you're making skin- and hair-care products. Turn to page 17 for how-tos.

2 tbsp	fresh or dried common mallow flowers (see tips, at left)	30 mL
4.6 oz	mineral water	130 g
4.2 oz	coco betaine (see tips, at left)	120 g
5	capsules borage oil (see tip, below), pierced and oil squeezed out	5
25	drops lavender essential oil	25

1. Place mallow flowers in a heatproof bowl. In a saucepan, bring mineral water to a boil. Pour boiling mineral water over mallow flowers. Cover and let steep for 10 minutes.

2. Using a fine-mesh sieve lined with cheesecloth, strain the mallow infusion into a clean bowl. Let cool completely.

3. Pour mallow infusion, coco betaine, borage oil and lavender essential oil into a bottle. Seal tightly. Shake gently to combine.

Tip: Borage oil capsules come in different dosages per capsule, which means the amount of oil you get from each one can vary. For this shampoo, the amount isn't as important, so you can just count out the capsules, pierce them and squeeze out the contents. If you're using a bottle of borage oil, this amount is between 0.07 and 0.1 oz (2 and 3 g).

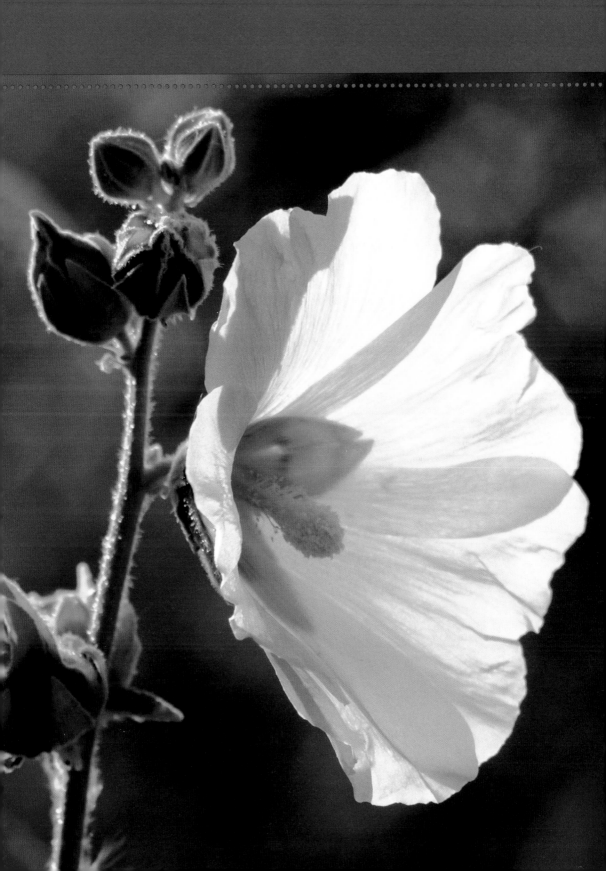

Borage Hair Repair Oil

A few drops of this woody-scented oil are enough to repair split ends. Place the oil on your fingertips and massage into the hair, concentrating on the ends.

Best for: Dry hair and split ends

Note: Exact measurements are important when you're making skin- and hair-care products. Turn to page 17 for how-tos.

0.35 oz	borage oil (about 20 capsules)	10 g
10	drops cedar essential oil (see tip, below)	10

1. Pour borage oil and cedar essential oil into a small glass bottle. Seal tightly.
2. Shake to combine.

Tip: The essential oils you use for skin- and hair-care products must be 100% pure. Don't use synthetic scents or oils, or essences designed for use in fragrance burners or lamp rings.

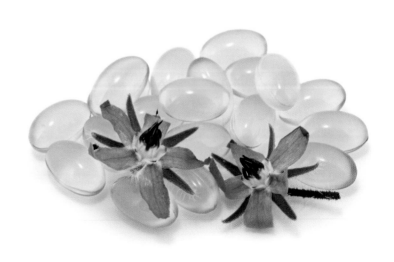

Borage and Peppermint Cream Conditioner

The zippy scent of peppermint livens up this rich, creamy conditioner and energizes you for the day ahead.

Best for: Dry to very dry hair

Tip: You can apply this conditioner to the ends alone or along the whole strand of hair; just avoid applying it directly to the scalp.

Note: Exact measurements are important when you're making skin- and hair-care products. Turn to page 17 for how-tos.

0.18 oz	borage oil (about 10 capsules)	5 g
0.15 oz	Lanette wax (see box, page 15)	4 g
6.5 oz	rose water (see tip, below)	185 g
2	pinches citric acid powder (see box, page 27)	2
2	pinches ascorbic acid powder	2
10	drops peppermint essential oil	10

1. Combine borage oil and Lanette wax in a saucepan. Heat over low heat just until ingredients are completely melted. Remove from heat and keep warm.

2. Pour rose water into a separate saucepan. Heat until lukewarm. Using a wooden spoon, stir in citric acid and ascorbic acid until dissolved.

3. Stir rose water mixture into oil mixture. Using a hand mixer, beat at low speed for 1 to 2 minutes. Let stand for 10 minutes.

4. Stir in peppermint essential oil. Using a hand mixer, beat at high speed for 1 minute.

5. Pour or spoon mixture into glass jars. Let cool.

Tip: Rose water is often used in Middle Eastern and Mediterranean cooking. Look for it in Middle Eastern grocery stores and some well-stocked supermarkets.

Borage Anti-Stretch Mark Cream

It is always better to prevent stretch marks rather than treat them after they appear, and this cream will help you do just that.

Best for: Areas prone to stretch marks, such as the belly, thighs and buttocks

Tips: Look for 100% pure beeswax that has been minimally processed. It is often sold in bulk, in chunks; if the recipe calls for a large amount, grate the wax so it will melt quickly and smoothly. Alternatively, you can buy beeswax that has been formed into pearls, which are easy to measure and melt quickly.

Stretch marks are always a possibility if you're pregnant or on a weight-loss regimen. During those times, apply the cream once a day, every day, for best results.

0.35 oz	borage oil (about 20 capsules)	10 g
0.35 oz	cocoa butter	10 g
0.2 oz	Lanette wax (see box, page 15)	6 g
0.1 oz	beeswax (see tips, at left)	3 g
5.6 oz	mineral water	160 g
2	pinches citric acid powder (see box, page 27)	2
2	pinches ascorbic acid powder	2
0.35 oz	rose hip seed oil	10 g

1. Combine borage oil, cocoa butter, Lanette wax and beeswax in a saucepan. Heat over low heat just until ingredients are completely melted. Remove from heat and keep warm.

2. Pour mineral water into a separate saucepan. Heat until lukewarm. Using a wooden spoon, stir in citric acid and ascorbic acid until dissolved.

3. Stir mineral water mixture into oil mixture. Using a hand mixer, beat at low speed for 1 to 2 minutes. Let stand for 10 minutes.

4. Stir in rose hip seed oil. Using a hand mixer, beat at high speed for 1 minute.

5. Pour or spoon mixture into glass jars. Let cool.

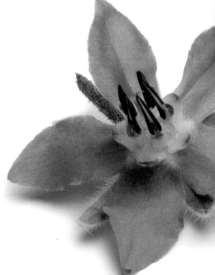

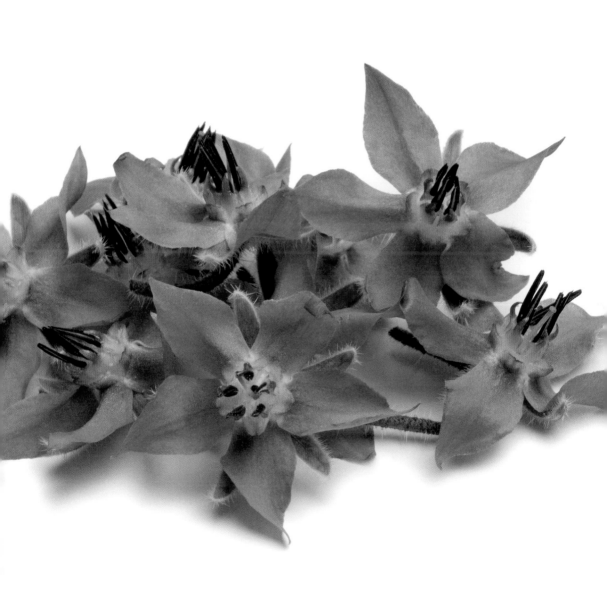

Borage and Jojoba Facial Oil

Mature skin needs a little TLC sometimes. Nourish it by applying a small amount of this oil to the face and gently massaging until it is completely absorbed.

Best for:
Mature skin

Tip: Store essential oils in a cool, dark place. Light exposure can diminish their healing properties.

Note: Exact measurements are important when you're making skin- and hair-care products. Turn to page 17 for how-tos.

0.35 oz	borage oil (about 20 capsules)	10 g
0.18 oz	jojoba oil	5 g
6	drops frankincense essential oil (see tip, at left)	6
6	drops myrrh essential oil	6
6	drops geranium essential oil	6

1. Pour borage oil, jojoba oil, and frankincense, myrrh and geranium essential oils into a small glass bottle. Seal tightly.

2. Shake to combine.

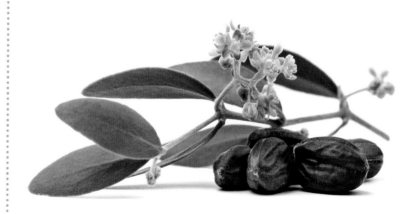

Borage and Wheat Germ Anti-Wrinkle Oil

Just a few drops of this emollient mixture smoothed over the face and neck are enough to bring quick results.

Best for:
Mature skin

Tips: You'll often find two types of chamomile essential oil at cosmetic-supply stores: German and Roman. They come from different strains of the chamomile plant, but both are soothing additions to homemade skin- and hair-care products.

The evergreen rosewood tree is an endangered and protected species in its native Brazil, so make sure you buy sustainably sourced rosewood essential oil. If you don't see any information on the label, ask the producer to disclose the source of the oil.

0.35 oz	wheat germ oil (see tip, below)	10 g
0.18 oz	borage oil (about 10 capsules)	5 g
4	drops chamomile essential oil (see tips, at left)	4
5	drops rosewood essential oil (see tips, at left)	5

1. Pour wheat germ oil, borage oil, and chamomile and rosewood essential oils into a small glass bottle. Seal tightly.

2. Shake to combine.

Tip: Wheat germ oil is highly perishable. Store it in the refrigerator to keep it from going rancid.

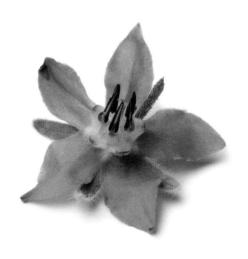

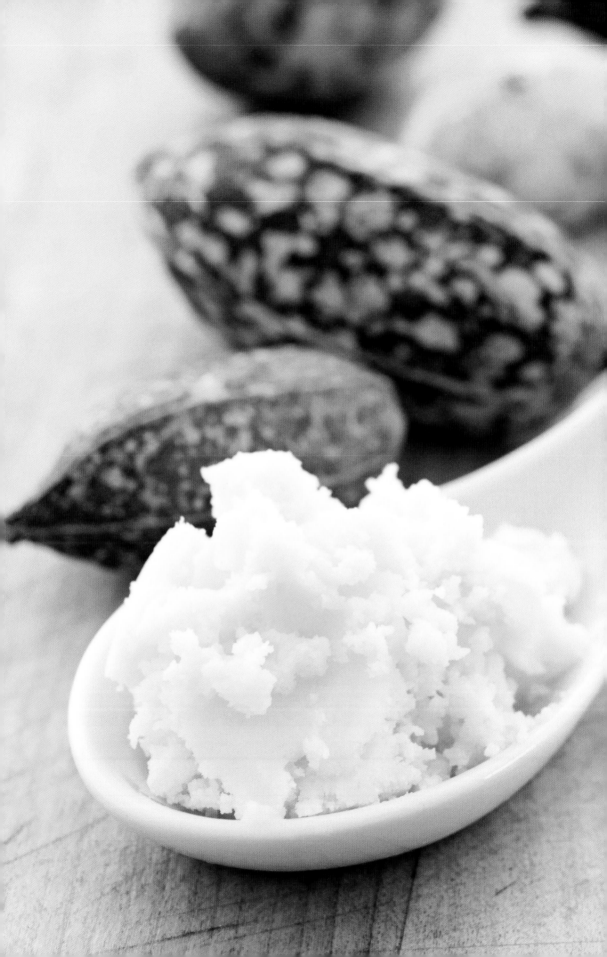

Shea Butter

Shea butter penetrates deeply to help heal cracked skin on the heels or hands. It's a terrific remedy for people who work outdoors.

Shea *(Vitellaria paradoxa),* also known as *Butyrospermum parkii* in skin- and hair-care formulas, is a tree that grows in the West African savanna. Its name means "butter tree," and it can live for up to 300 years.

Since ancient times, Africans have cooked the pulp and peel of the shea nut for food. Shea butter is extracted from the seeds by pressing; it is used in both food and cosmetics. In Senegal's salty Lac Rose (Pink Lake), workers collect salt by hand, an arduous and skin-drying job. They rub their bodies with shea butter (called *beurre de karité* in French) to protect their skin.

Shea butter is an excellent natural cell regenerator that prevents aging of the skin and hair. It softens the skin, fights wrinkles and protects the skin from the sun and cold. It is rich in vitamin E, stearic acid, oleic acid, linoleic acid and catechins.

Pure shea butter comes in chunks, like cocoa butter, at cosmetic-supply stores. Break or chop it up before adding it to the other ingredients in the oil-based portion of cream recipes. The smaller pieces will melt quickly and easily.

Shea Butter Moisturizing Anti-Wrinkle Cream

This cream is wonderful for preventing wrinkles, and for treating them once they have appeared.

Best for: Dry skin, or skin that's just starting to wrinkle

Note: Exact measurements are important when you're making skin- and hair-care products. Turn to page 17 for how-tos.

1 oz	shea butter	30 g
0.2 oz	Lanette wax (see box, page 15)	6 g
5.5 oz	mineral water	155 g
2	pinches citric acid powder (see box, page 27)	2
2	pinches ascorbic acid powder	2
0.35 oz	rose hip seed oil	10 g
15	drops orange essential oil	15

1. Combine shea butter and Lanette wax in a saucepan. Heat over low heat just until ingredients are completely melted. Remove from heat and keep warm.

2. Pour mineral water into a separate saucepan. Heat until lukewarm. Using a wooden spoon, stir in citric acid and ascorbic acid until dissolved.

3. Stir mineral water mixture into oil mixture. Using a hand mixer, beat at low speed for 1 to 2 minutes. Let stand for 10 minutes.

4. Stir in rose hip seed oil and orange essential oil. Using a hand mixer, beat at high speed for 1 minute.

5. Pour or spoon mixture into glass jars. Let cool.

Shea Butter Prevents Pregnancy-Related Stretch Marks

As the body grows during pregnancy, stretch marks may appear on the belly and breasts. But you can use shea butter to prevent them. Every day, spread 100% pure shea butter on the breasts and abdomen, gently massaging to allow the oil to penetrate the skin. Don't add anything to the shea butter — pregnant women should be very careful to use simple, pure body-care products.

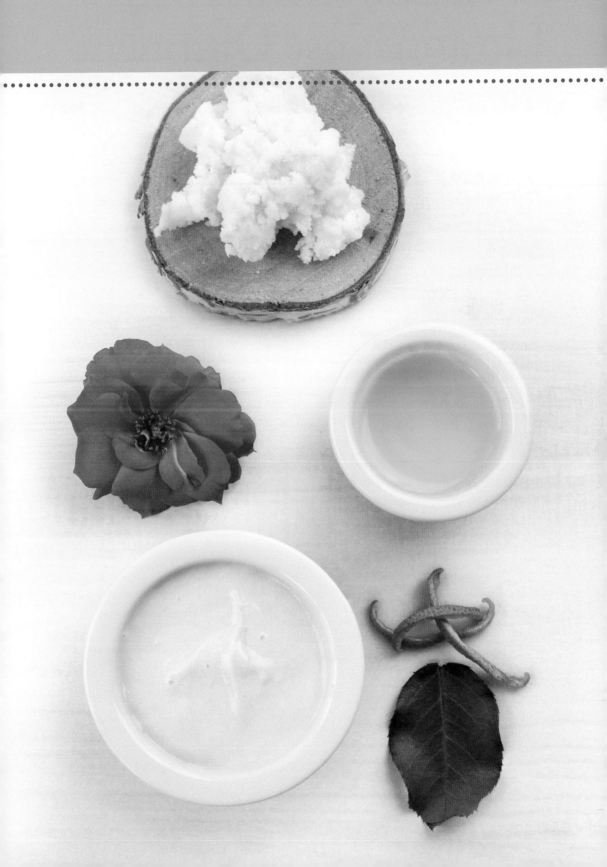

Shea Butter Chapped Lip and Nose Ointment

This ointment is great for treating the customary chapped lips and nose that accompany a cold. A small amount applied regularly will solve the problem.

Best for: Sore, chapped lips and nose

Note: Exact measurements are important when you're making skin- and hair-care products. Turn to page 17 for how-tos.

| 1 oz | shea butter | 30 g |
| 10 | drops bergamot essential oil | 10 |

1. In a saucepan, heat shea butter over low heat just until completely melted.

2. Stir in bergamot essential oil. Pour mixture into a small glass jar. Seal tightly.

3. Let cool.

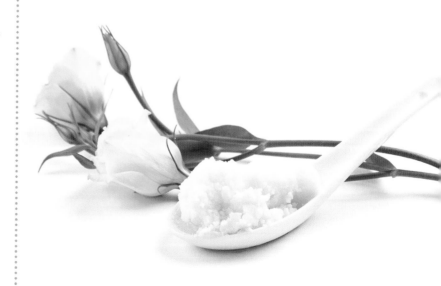

Shea Butter Corn and Callus Ointment

Calluses and their painful cousins, corns, are built-up areas of tissue that form where the skin of the foot is constantly rubbed or pressed. This soothing cream helps heal and repair them.

Best for: Corns and calluses

Tip: For relief from these painful foot problems, spread a generous layer of this ointment over the area to be treated, cover with gauze and leave overnight. The skin will soften up, and the pain will diminish.

Note: Exact measurements are important when you're making skin- and hair-care products. Turn to page 17 for how-tos.

1.8 oz	shea butter	50 g
20	drops cedar essential oil	20
10	drops myrrh essential oil	10

1. In a saucepan, heat shea butter over low heat just until completely melted.

2. Stir in cedar and myrrh essential oils. Pour mixture into a small glass jar. Seal tightly.

3. Let cool.

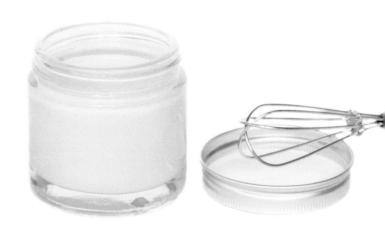

Shea Butter Ointment for Cracked Heels

Cracked skin on your heels can really hurt, and it can be hard to repair. But if you apply a generous amount of this ointment, then cover your feet with cotton socks overnight, you'll soon see amazing results.

Best for: Cracked skin on the heels

Note: Exact measurements are important when you're making skin- and hair-care products. Turn to page 17 for how-tos.

1.8 oz	shea butter	50 g
10	drops cypress essential oil	10
10	drops tea tree essential oil (see tip, below)	10

1. In a saucepan, heat shea butter over low heat just until completely melted.

2. Stir in cypress and tea tree essential oils. Pour mixture into a small glass jar. Seal tightly.

3. Let cool.

Tip: Tea tree essential oil has potent antibacterial and antifungal powers. It is an excellent addition to this ointment because it keeps painful cracks from becoming infected and inflamed.

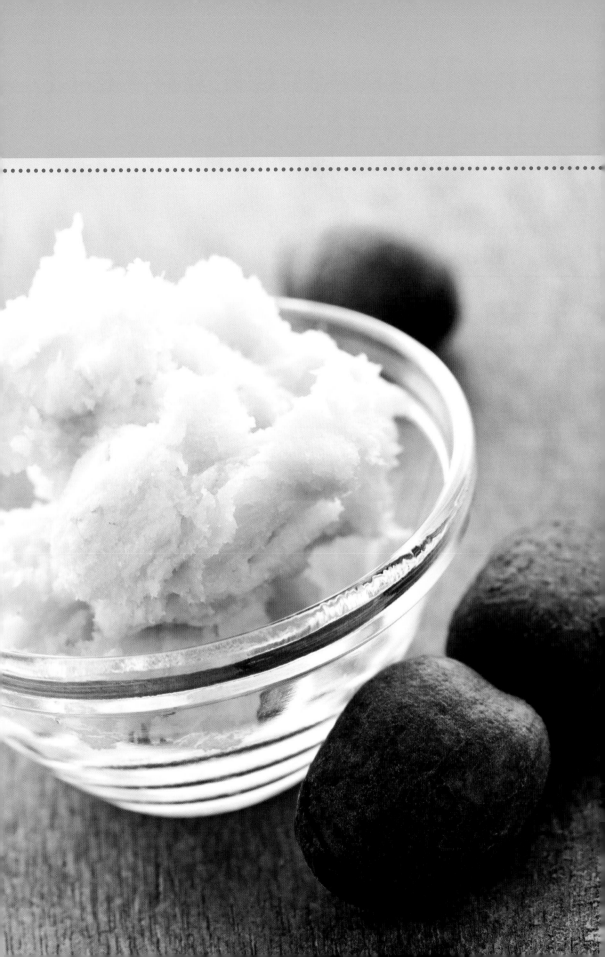

Shea Butter and Citronella Mosquito Repellent

Scare away mosquitoes naturally. Rub a small amount of this ointment in your hands until warm and spread all over your body to prevent bites.

Best for: All skin types

Tip: Citronella essential oil has a strong lemongrass-like aroma. It's often used in perfumes, and is a natural insect repellent.

Note: Exact measurements are important when you're making skin- and hair-care products. Turn to page 17 for how-tos.

| 1.8 oz | shea butter | 50 g |
| 30 | drops citronella essential oil (see tip, at left) | 30 |

1. In a saucepan, heat shea butter over low heat just until completely melted.

2. Stir in citronella essential oil. Pour mixture into a small glass jar. Seal tightly.

3. Let cool.

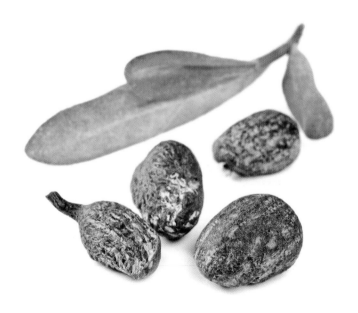

Shea Butter Joint-Pain Ointment

Ease the discomfort of stiff, painful joints by massaging in this ointment, using light but swift movements. Warm it up first to intensify the action.

Best for: Achy, sore joints

Tip: You'll often find two types of chamomile essential oil at cosmetic-supply stores: German and Roman. They come from different strains of the chamomile plant, but both are soothing additions to homemade skin- and hair-care products.

Note: Exact measurements are important when you're making skin- and hair-care products. Turn to page 17 for how-tos.

Caution: Do not use rosemary essential oil if you have epilepsy or high blood pressure.

3.5 oz	shea butter	100 g
20	drops ginger essential oil	20
20	drops rosemary essential oil (see caution, at left)	20
20	drops chamomile essential oil (see tip, at left)	20

1. In a saucepan, heat shea butter over low heat just until completely melted.

2. Stir in ginger, rosemary and chamomile essential oils. Pour mixture into a small glass jar. Seal tightly.

3. Let cool.

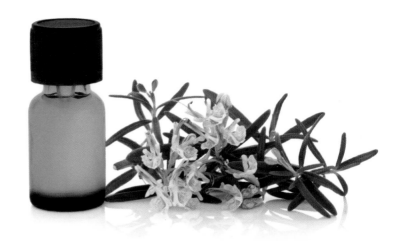

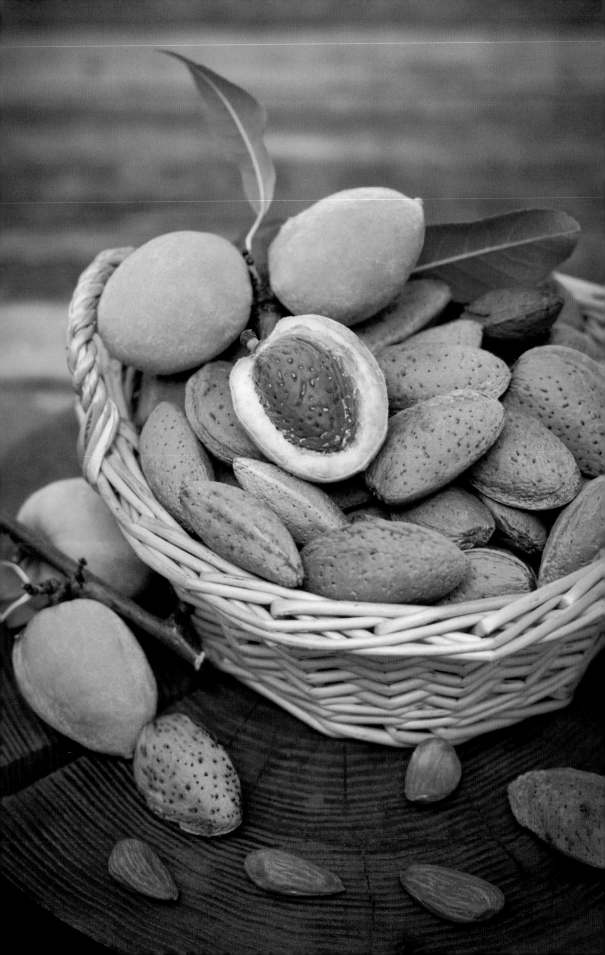

Bitter Almond Oil

Bitter almond oil has been used extensively throughout the ages by all of the great Mediterranean civilizations.

Bitter almond *(Amygdalus communis* var. *amara* or *Prunus amygdalus* var. *amara)* has been used since ancient times to make liquors and other beverages. It is also used in small doses to make traditional remedies. The oil is made from a different variety of almond than sweet almond oil, which is also used in skin-care formulas. They are not interchangeable in recipes.

The scent of bitter almond oil is well known around the world, because marzipan candies contain a small amount of bitter almond extract, which gives them their characteristic aroma and flavor. The substance that gives the oil its distinctive fragrance is a compound called amygdalin, while the flavor is created by hydrocyanic acid, which is poisonous if consumed in large amounts.

Bitter almond oil has a number of beneficial skin-care properties that make it ideal for use in homemade body-care products. For example, it softens the skin and makes it smooth and flexible. The oil can also be used as a remedy for sunburns and to eliminate freckles and blemishes.

Almond-Apricot Massage Oil

To apply, pour a bit of this luxurious oil in the palm of your hand, spread it over both hands and massage into tired muscles.

Best for: All skin types

| 3.5 oz | apricot kernel oil (see tip, below) | 100 g |
| 0.7 oz | bitter almond oil | 20 g |

1. Pour apricot kernel oil and bitter almond oil into a small glass bottle. Seal tightly.

2. Shake to combine.

Tip: Choose extra-virgin or virgin oils made from the first cold pressing.

Bitter Almond Moisturizing Oil

Applied after an exfoliation session, this oil will leave your skin incredibly soft and smooth.

Best for:
Replenishing skin after exfoliation

Note: Exact measurements are important when you're making skin- and hair-care products. Turn to page 17 for how-tos.

1.8 oz	jojoba oil	50 g
0.35 oz	bitter almond oil	10 g
10	drops geranium essential oil (see tip, below)	10

1. Pour jojoba oil, bitter almond oil and geranium essential oil into a small glass bottle. Seal tightly.

2. Shake to combine.

Tip: The essential oils you use for skin- and hair-care products must be 100% pure. Don't use synthetic scents or oils, or essences used in fragrance burners or lamp rings.

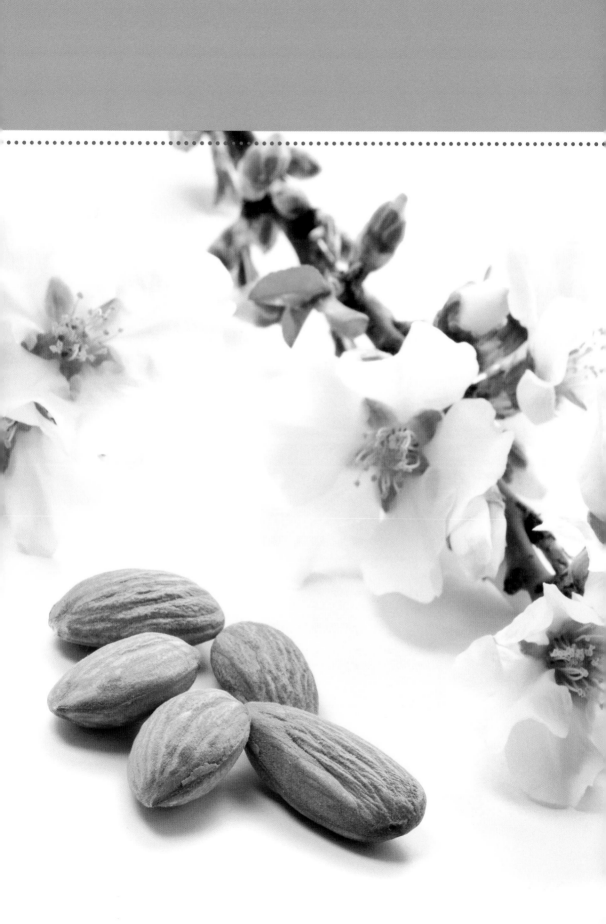

Bitter Almond Freckle- and Spot-Removing Oil

This oil will reduce the appearance of freckles and spots, and lighten your overall skin tone. Moisten a cotton ball with it and apply gently to skin once or twice a day. Close the bottle tightly after each use.

Best for: Lightening skin tones, blemishes and freckles

Tip: Look for mother-of-pearl or pearl powder at cosmetic-supply stores. It does double-duty as a moisturizing and skin-lightening ingredient.

Note: Exact measurements are important when you're making skin- and hair-care products. Turn to page 17 for how-tos.

0.5 oz	bitter almond oil	15 g
0.35 oz	castor oil	10 g
0.07 oz	mother-of-pearl powder or pearl powder (see tip, at left)	2 g

1. Pour bitter almond oil, castor oil and mother-of-pearl powder into a small glass bottle. Seal tightly.

2. Shake to combine.

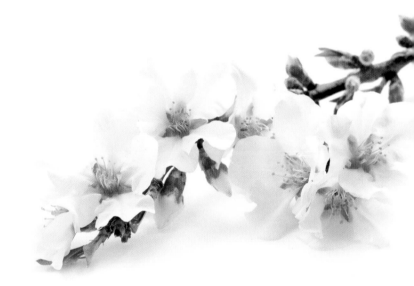

Bitter Almond Sunburn Relief Oil

Feeling the burn? Gently smooth this oil over sunburned skin, repeating the treatment every eight hours if the sensation is intense.

Best for:
Sunburned skin

Tips: Choose extra-virgin or virgin oils made from the first cold pressing.

Store the finished oil away from light to keep its healing properties intact. This is a smart policy for all homemade oils.

Note: Exact measurements are important when you're making skin- and hair-care products. Turn to page 17 for how-tos.

0.7 oz	bitter almond oil	20 g
0.7 oz	olive oil (see tips, at left)	20 g
20	drops marjoram essential oil	20
20	drops lavender essential oil	20

1. Pour bitter almond oil, olive oil, and marjoram and lavender essential oils into a small glass bottle. Seal tightly.

2. Shake to combine.

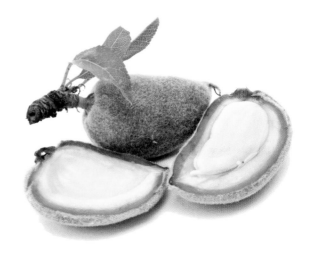

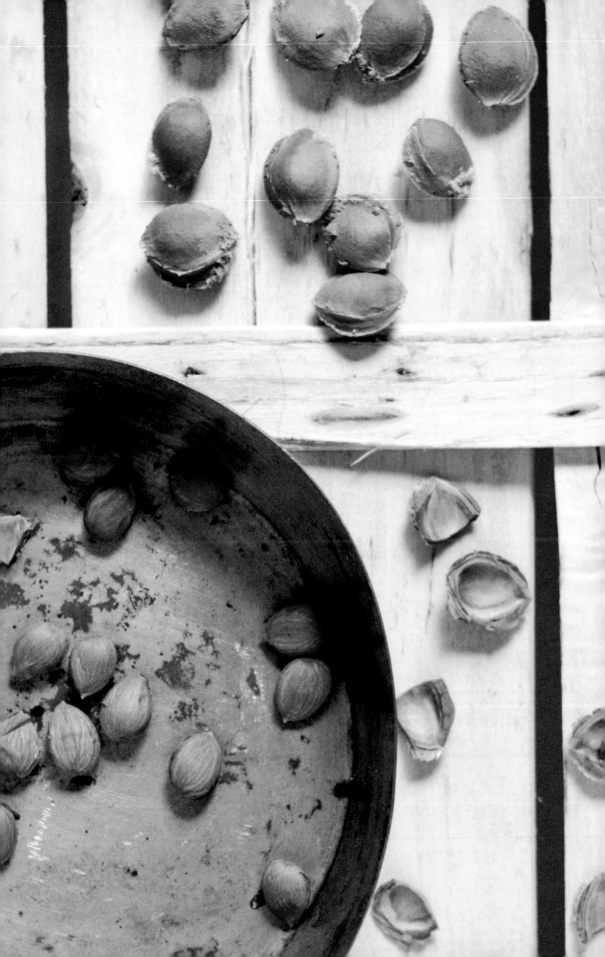

Apricot Kernel Oil

Apricot kernel oil has a neutral scent that does not alter the fragrances of essential oils.

The apricot tree *(Prunus armeniaca)* belongs to the Rosaceae family and is thought to be native to Asia (possibly to China), though its specific origin is not entirely certain. The oil extracted from the pits (or kernels) inside the fruit is very light and quickly absorbed by the skin, making it excellent for use in cosmetics.

Apricot kernel oil has many beneficial skin-care properties. It contains a high concentration of vitamins A and E, monounsaturated fatty acids (including omega-9 oleic acid) and polyunsaturated fatty acids (including omega-6 linoleic acid). Apricot kernel oil is quite resistant to spoilage, as it contains a large amount of carotenes and antioxidant vitamins, which act as natural preservatives.

Although this valued oil has been known for centuries, it is not among the most popular oils in skin-care formulas (though it should be, given its usefulness). It regenerates tired-looking skin and soothes sensitive skin. It restores softness and elasticity, as well. Another of its interesting benefits is that it relieves irritation from shaving. And it is one of the most suitable oils for the sensitive skin of children and the elderly. Furthermore, it is one of the best base oils in which to dissolve essential oils because it does not alter their natural aromas.

Apricot Kernel Moisturizing Face Cream

Supremely gentle, this cream is the perfect hydrating formula for people with delicate skin.

Best for: Sensitive skin, especially in children and the elderly

Tip: Pure shea butter comes in chunks, like cocoa butter, at cosmetic-supply stores. Break or chop it up before adding it to the saucepan so that it melts quickly and easily.

Note: Exact measurements are important when you're making skin- and hair-care products. Turn to page 17 for how-tos.

1 oz	apricot kernel oil	30 g
0.2 oz	Lanette wax (see box, page 15)	6 g
0.18 oz	shea butter (see tip, at left)	5 g
5.6 oz	mineral water	160 g
2	pinches citric acid powder (see box, page 27)	2
2	pinches ascorbic acid powder	2
12	drops lavender essential oil	12

1. Combine apricot kernel oil, Lanette wax and shea butter in a saucepan. Heat over low heat just until ingredients are completely melted. Remove from heat and keep warm.

2. Pour mineral water into a separate saucepan. Heat until lukewarm. Using a wooden spoon, stir in citric acid and ascorbic acid until dissolved.

3. Stir mineral water mixture into oil mixture. Using a hand mixer, beat at low speed for 1 to 2 minutes. Let stand for 10 minutes.

4. Stir in lavender essential oil. Using a hand mixer, beat at high speed for 1 minute.

5. Pour or spoon mixture into glass jars. Let cool.

Apricot Kernel Oil: An Ideal Cleanser

Apricot kernel oil on its own is an excellent cleanser for the face and under the eyes. It works whether you are wearing makeup or not — it cleanses bare skin and easily removes makeup, too. For best results, moisten a cotton pad with a bit of water, then squeeze out excess water firmly between your palms. Add a few drops of apricot kernel oil to the pad and gently rub over your skin. Use a second cotton pad, prepared the same way, to remove eye makeup.

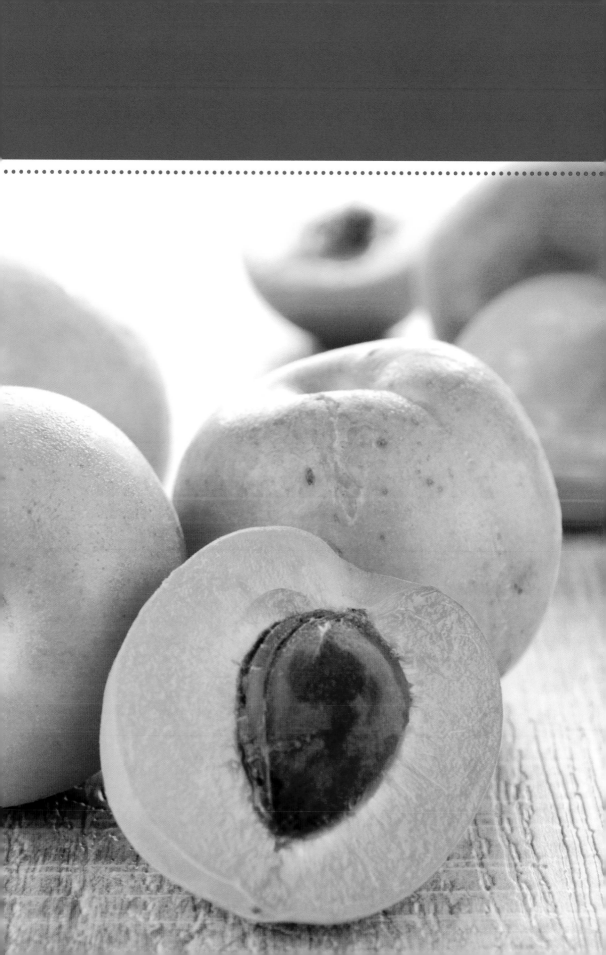

Apricot Kernel Moisturizing Body Cream

Kids and seniors often suffer from dry skin all over their bodies. Daily moisturizing with this formula will help soften and hydrate the skin.

Best for: Sensitive skin, especially in children and the elderly

Tips: Rose water is often used in Middle Eastern and Mediterranean cooking. Look for it in Middle Eastern grocery stores and some well-stocked supermarkets.

Look for pure vitamin E in liquid form at cosmetic-supply stores. It's also easy to buy online.

Note: Exact measurements are important when you're making skin- and hair-care products. Turn to page 17 for how-tos.

1.4 oz	apricot kernel oil	40 g
0.4 oz	Lanette wax (see box, page 15)	12 g
0.35 oz	cocoa butter	10 g
11.8 oz	rose water (see tips, at left)	335 g
4	pinches citric acid powder (see box, page 27)	4
4	pinches ascorbic acid powder	4
0.18 oz	pure vitamin E (see tips, at left)	5 g
10	drops frankincense essential oil	10

1. Combine apricot kernel oil, Lanette wax and cocoa butter in a saucepan. Heat over low heat just until ingredients are completely melted. Remove from heat and keep warm.

2. Pour rose water into a separate saucepan. Heat until lukewarm. Using a wooden spoon, stir in citric acid and ascorbic acid until dissolved.

3. Stir rose water mixture into oil mixture. Using a hand mixer, beat at low speed for 1 to 2 minutes. Let stand for 10 minutes.

4. Stir in vitamin E and frankincense essential oil. Using a hand mixer, beat at high speed for 1 minute.

5. Pour or spoon mixture into glass jars. Let cool.

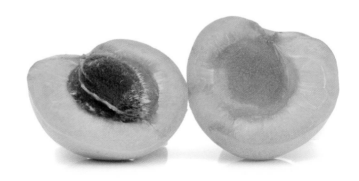

Apricot Kernel Super Moisturizing Cream

This ultra-rich cream is especially recommended for areas where the skin is dry and flaky.

Best for: Sensitive skin, especially in children and the elderly

Tips: Lanolin is a waxy natural moisturizer derived from sheep's wool. It has long been used as a softening and moisturizing agent, especially in hand creams. You can find jars of it at cosmetic-supply stores. It has a distinctive, earthy aroma, and a little goes a long way.

Orange flower water is also called orange blossom water. It's easy to find in Middle Eastern grocery stores and some well-stocked supermarkets, where it's sold for use in cooking.

1 oz	apricot kernel oil	30 g
0.35 oz	shea butter	10 g
0.2 oz	Lanette wax (see box, page 15)	6 g
0.15 oz	lanolin (see tips, at left)	4 g
5.3 oz	orange flower water (see tips, at left)	150 g
2	pinches citric acid powder (see box, page 27)	2
2	pinches ascorbic acid powder	2
10	drops frankincense essential oil	10

1. Combine apricot kernel oil, shea butter, Lanette wax and lanolin in a saucepan. Heat over low heat just until ingredients are completely melted. Remove from heat and keep warm.

2. Pour orange flower water into a separate saucepan. Heat until lukewarm. Using a wooden spoon, stir in citric acid and ascorbic acid until dissolved.

3. Stir orange flower water mixture into oil mixture. Using a hand mixer, beat at low speed for 1 to 2 minutes. Let stand for 10 minutes.

4. Stir in frankincense essential oil. Using a hand mixer, beat at high speed for 1 minute.

5. Pour or spoon mixture into glass jars. Let cool.

Apricot Kernel Scrub for Sensitive Skin

Apply this scrub anywhere that needs exfoliating, including the face. It's gentle but effective.

Best for:
Sensitive skin

Tip: Apricot kernel meal is just finely ground apricot kernels. Look for packages of this convenient additive in cosmetic-supply stores. The kernels are quite hard, so it's easier not to grind them yourself.

Note: Exact measurements are important when you're making skin- and hair-care products.

Turn to page 17 for how-tos.

| 1.6 oz | apricot kernel meal (see tip, at left) | 45 g |
| 0.7 oz | apricot kernel oil | 20 g |

1. Combine apricot kernel meal and oil in a bowl.

2. Using a wooden spoon, stir until ingredients are well combined. Use immediately.

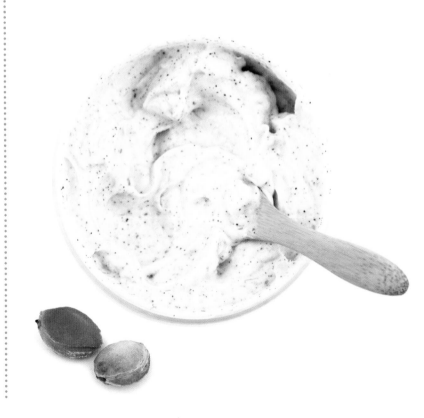

Apricot Kernel Diaper Rash Cream

Babies will soon find relief when you apply this cream to areas affected by diaper rash. It gets irritated skin back to normal.

Best for:
Diaper rash

Tip: Calendulas are also known as marigolds, and they are excellent at healing wounds and skin irritations. They're also easy to grow, so plant some in the spring and enjoy the blooms both in the garden and in your homemade skin-care formulas. Alternatively, herbalists' shops often carry the dried flowers.

Note: Exact measurements are important when you're making skin- and hair-care products. Turn to page 17 for how-tos.

3 tbsp	fresh or dried calendula petals (see tip, at left)	45 mL
4.8 oz	mineral water	135 g
2	pinches citric acid powder (see box, page 27)	2
2	pinches ascorbic acid powder	2
1.4 oz	apricot kernel oil	40 g
0.35 oz	shea butter	10 g
0.2 oz	Lanette wax (see box, page 15)	6 g
0.18 oz	lanolin	5 g
0.15 oz	beeswax (see tip, below)	4 g

1. Place calendula petals in a heatproof bowl. In a saucepan, bring mineral water to a boil. Pour boiling mineral water over calendula petals. Cover and let steep for 10 minutes.

2. Using a fine-mesh sieve lined with cheesecloth, strain the calendula infusion into a clean bowl. Let cool until lukewarm. Using a wooden spoon, stir in citric acid and ascorbic acid until dissolved. Keep warm.

3. Combine apricot kernel oil, shea butter, Lanette wax, lanolin and beeswax in a separate saucepan. Heat over low heat just until ingredients are completely melted. Remove from heat.

4. Stir calendula infusion mixture into oil mixture. Using a hand mixer, beat at low speed for 1 to 2 minutes. Let stand for 10 minutes.

5. Using a hand mixer, beat at high speed for 1 minute. Pour or spoon mixture into glass jars. Let cool.

Tip: Look for 100% pure beeswax that has been minimally processed. It is often sold in bulk, in chunks; if the recipe calls for a large amount, grate the wax so it will melt quickly and smoothly. Alternatively, you can buy beeswax that has been formed into pearls, which are easy to measure and melt quickly.

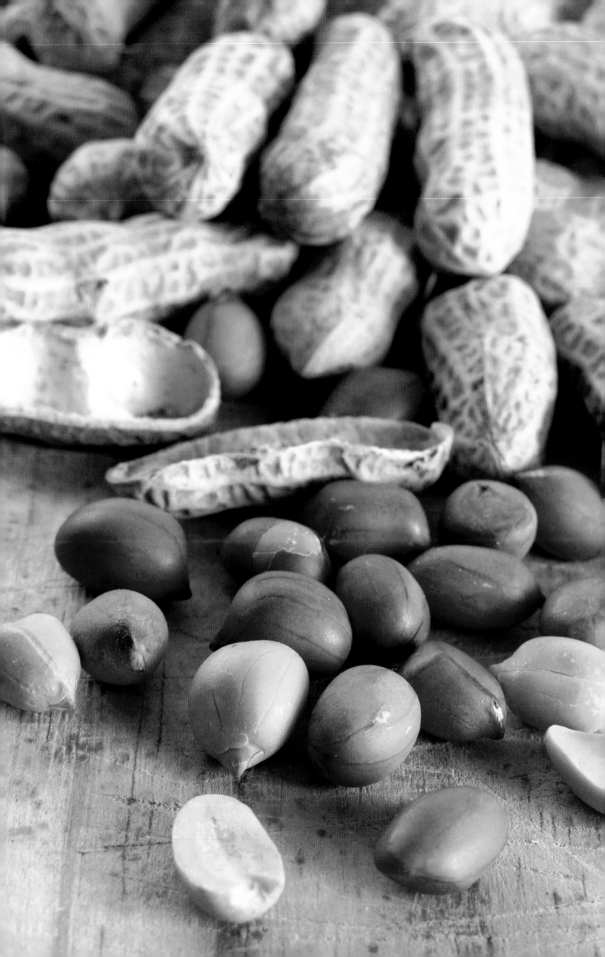

Peanut Oil

Peanut oil is well known and loved as a cooking oil, but it is also excellent at hydrating and repairing dry skin.

The peanut plant *(Arachis hypogaea)* is a legume that belongs to the family Fabaceae. It is also known by other common names, including groundnut, goober pea, earthnut and monkey nut. Its origin is likely Peru or Brazil, but it is now grown in many places around the world.

Peanut oil is obtained from the well-known fruit of the plant, which grows underground. Like olive oil, peanut oil is rich in fatty acids, mainly omega-9 oleic acid. It is used as an ingredient in cooking and is popular in North and South America, and Asia, where it appears in countless recipes.

Peanut oil serves as the base of all sorts of ointments, liniments, soaps and other products. It is well suited for making ointments and creams for very dry skin. The oil has long been used to repair brittle, dry nails, as well.

Store peanut oil in a cool place away from light. When exposed to the air excessively, the oil will thicken and become rancid, so keep the bottle tightly sealed. If it becomes rancid, it will develop an unpleasant odor, though it will not lose its beneficial qualities. If it's stored in the refrigerator, peanut oil will solidify, but it can be melted over low heat and used without any problem.

Peanut Ointment for Rough Hands

The most effective way to use this cream is to slather a generous amount onto your hands and slip on cotton gloves for an overnight softening treatment.

Best for: Rough, damaged skin on the hands

Tip: Look for 100% pure beeswax that has been minimally processed. It is often sold in bulk, in chunks; if the recipe calls for a large amount, grate the wax so it will melt quickly and smoothly. Alternatively, you can buy beeswax that has been formed into pearls, which are easy to measure and melt quickly.

Note: Exact measurements are important when you're making skin- and hair-care products. Turn to page 17 for how-tos.

1 oz	peanut oil	30 g
0.35 oz	cocoa butter	10 g
0.2 oz	Lanette wax (see box, page 15)	6 g
0.18 oz	beeswax (see tip, at left)	5 g
4.6 oz	mineral water	130 g
2	pinches citric acid powder (see box, page 27)	2
2	pinches ascorbic acid powder	2
0.35 oz	liquid glycerin	10 g
0.35 oz	soluble collagen (see tip, below)	10 g
10	drops sandalwood essential oil	10

1. Combine peanut oil, cocoa butter, Lanette wax and beeswax in a saucepan. Heat over low heat just until ingredients are completely melted. Remove from heat and keep warm.

2. Pour mineral water into a separate saucepan. Heat until lukewarm. Using a wooden spoon, stir in citric acid and ascorbic acid until dissolved.

3. Stir mineral water mixture into oil mixture. Using a hand mixer, beat at low speed for 1 to 2 minutes. Let stand for 10 minutes.

4. Stir in glycerin, collagen and sandalwood essential oil. Using a hand mixer, beat at high speed for 1 minute.

5. Pour or spoon mixture into glass jars. Let cool.

Tip: Soluble collagen is a moisturizing ingredient that is often added to cosmetics. It comes in powder form at cosmetic-supply stores.

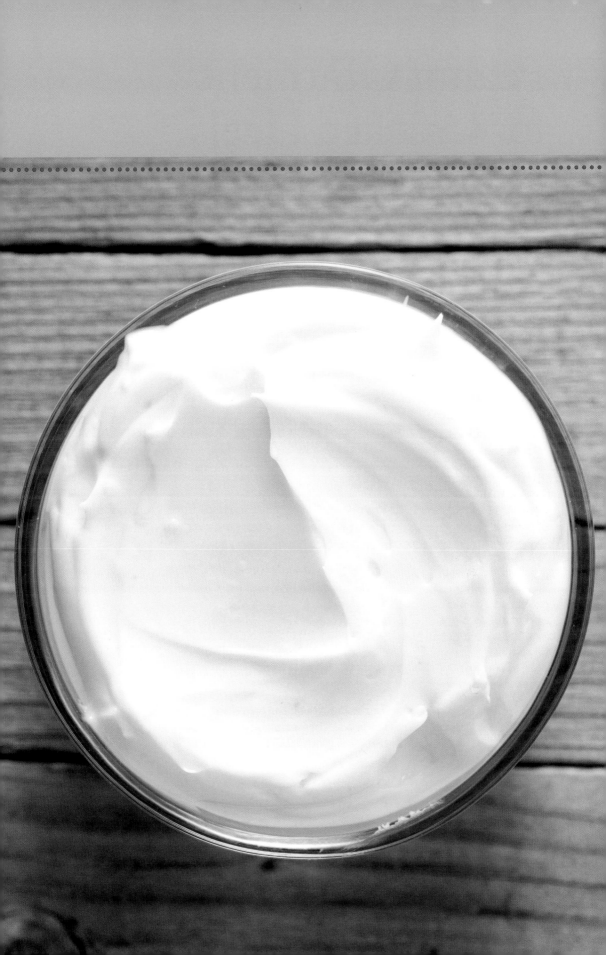

Peanut Ointment for Cracked Heels

Cracked heels and feet really hurt. Get quick relief by applying a generous amount of this ointment to your feet and covering them with cotton socks overnight.

Best for: Very dry feet and cracked skin on the heels

Tip: Lanolin is a waxy natural moisturizer derived from sheep's wool. It has long been used as a softening and moisturizing agent, especially in hand creams. You can find jars of it at cosmetic-supply stores. It has a distinctive, earthy aroma, and a little goes a long way.

Note: Exact measurements are important when you're making skin- and hair-care products. Turn to page 17 for how-tos.

1 oz	peanut oil	30 g
0.7 oz	lanolin (see tip, at left)	20 g
0.35 oz	shea butter (see tips, below)	10 g
0.2 oz	Lanette wax (see box, page 15)	6 g
0.18 oz	beeswax	5 g
4.4 oz	witch hazel	125 g
2	pinches citric acid powder (see box, page 27)	2
2	pinches ascorbic acid powder	2
0.15 oz	pure vitamin A (see tips, below)	4 g
10	drops bergamot essential oil	10

1. Combine peanut oil, lanolin, shea butter, Lanette wax and beeswax in a saucepan. Heat over low heat just until ingredients are completely melted. Remove from heat and keep warm.

2. Pour witch hazel into a separate saucepan. Heat until lukewarm. Using a wooden spoon, stir in citric acid and ascorbic acid until dissolved.

3. Stir witch hazel mixture into oil mixture. Using a hand mixer, beat at low speed for 1 to 2 minutes. Let stand for 10 minutes.

4. Stir in vitamin A and bergamot essential oil. Using a hand mixer, beat at high speed for 1 minute.

5. Pour or spoon mixture into glass jars. Let cool.

Tips: Pure shea butter comes in chunks, like cocoa butter, at cosmetic-supply stores. Break or chop it up before adding it to the saucepan so that it melts quickly and easily.

Look for pure vitamin A in liquid form at cosmetic-supply stores. It's also easy to buy online.

Peanut Facial Oil

Banish dry patches and flaky skin with this rich facial oil. Place a few drops on your fingertips and spread over your face and neck.

Best for: Dry, flaky skin on the face

Tip: You'll often find two types of chamomile essential oil at cosmetic-supply stores: German and Roman. They come from different strains of the chamomile plant, but both are soothing additions to homemade skin- and hair-care products.

Note: Exact measurements are important when you're making skin- and hair-care products. Turn to page 17 for how-tos.

0.7 oz	peanut oil	20 g
0.35 oz	St. John's wort oil	10 g
10	drops myrrh essential oil	10
10	drops chamomile essential oil (see tip, at left)	10

1. Pour peanut oil, St. John's wort oil, and myrrh and chamomile essential oils into a small glass bottle. Seal tightly.

2. Shake to combine.

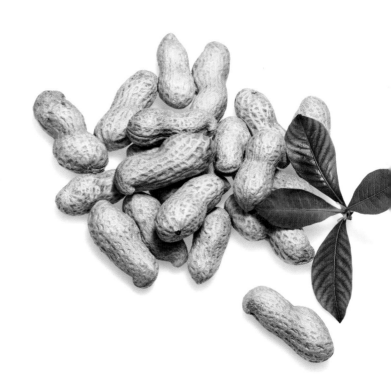

Peanut Moisturizing Body Oil

With a lemony scent and a smooth, moisturizing oil base, this treatment is a pleasant way to hydrate dried-out skin all over your body.

Best for: Dry skin

5.3 oz	peanut oil	150 g
0.9 oz	walnut oil	25 g
10	drops citronella essential oil (see tips, below)	10

1. Pour peanut oil, walnut oil and citronella essential oil into a small glass bottle. Seal tightly.

2. Shake to combine.

Tips: Citronella essential oil has a strong lemongrass-like aroma. It's often used in perfumes, and is a natural insect repellent.

You can make applying this oil very convenient if you pour it into a bottle with a roll-on top.

Peanut Nail-Strengthening Oil

This oil will have your nails in top shape in no time. It makes an excellent pampering treatment while still warm (see tips, at right).

Best for: Fragile, split nails

| 1 oz | peanut oil | 30 g |
| 1 oz | olive oil (see tips, below) | 30 g |

1. Pour peanut and olive oils into a small saucepan.

2. Heat over low heat until warm. Use immediately.

Tips: Choose extra-virgin or virgin oils made from the first cold pressing.

While the oil is still warm, submerge the nails on one hand in the mixture and let soak for 15 minutes. Repeat with the other hand, rewarming the oil slightly if necessary. Wipe the oil off with a cotton ball and avoid wetting your hands for two hours.

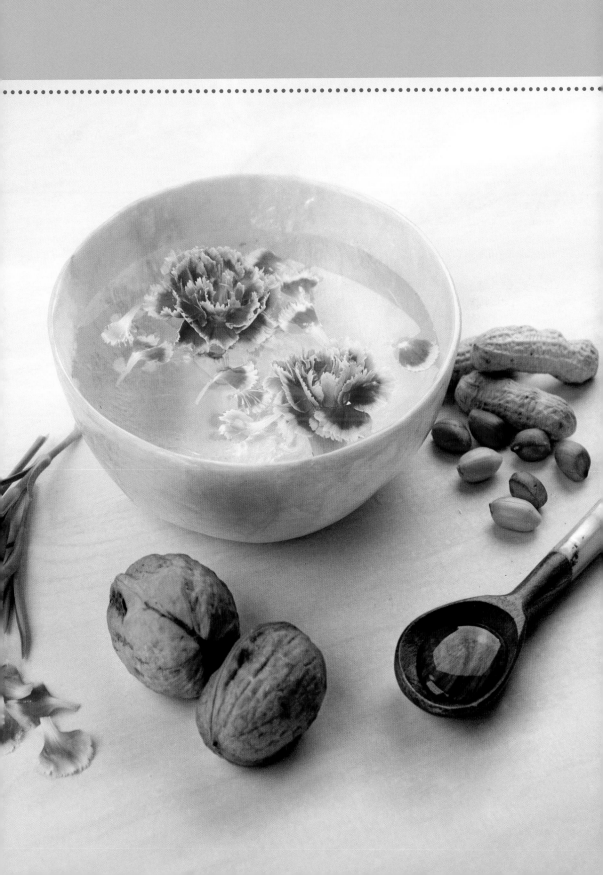

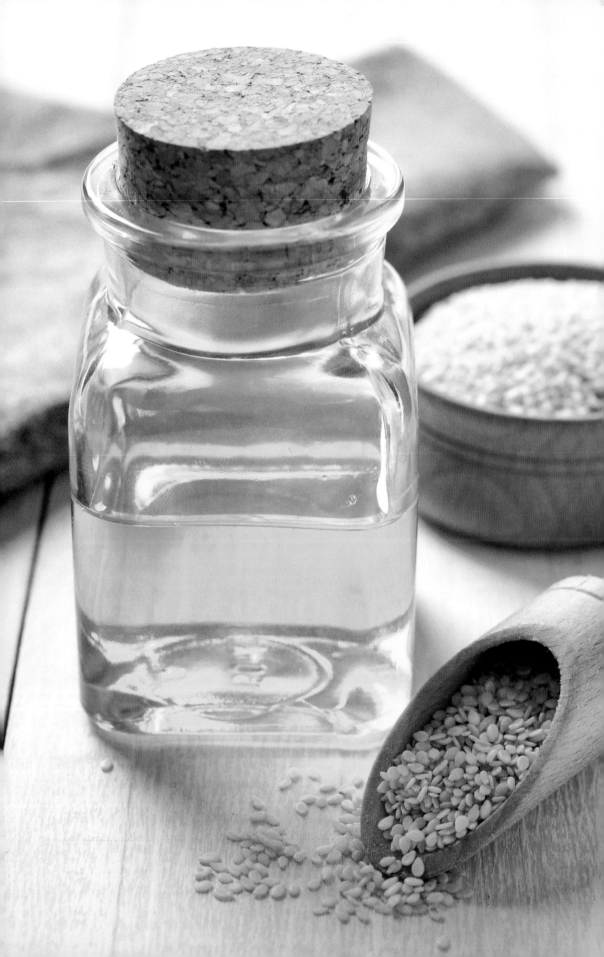

Sesame Oil

In Ayurvedic treatments, sesame oil is warmed slightly before use, because the warm oil produces deep relaxation.

Remember the famous phrase "Open Sesame!" from the story "Ali Baba and the 40 Thieves"? In the story, it was a secret password that opened the door to a cave full of riches. But we can take it a little more literally. Sesame oil has healing properties and strengthens the nervous system. If we open the sesame seed and extract its oil, we are opening the door to good health and better immunity to illness.

This prized oil is extracted from the seeds of the sesame plant *(Sesamum indicum)*. Sesame was one of the first plants from which humans extracted oil. Indeed, in Hindi, the word for "oil" is derived from the word for "sesame."

Sesame oil is widely used in cooking in India, South Korea, China and Japan. It is rich in fatty acids, especially polyunsaturated omega-6 and monounsaturated omega-9 fatty acids. The oil also contains large amounts of vitamins E and K, and folic acid. Sesame oil is prized for its mineral content; it offers calcium, magnesium, potassium and iron.

In addition to its usefulness as a cooking oil, sesame oil nourishes the skin magnificently, making it desirable in cosmetic formulas. The most healing option is to consume it in food and use it externally, to nourish the skin from the inside and the outside at the same time. A curious fact about sesame oil is that massaging a little bit of it onto cold feet in winter will keep them warm all day.

Sesame Relaxing Oil

The natural warming powers of sesame oil mean this formula is tailor-made for a wonderful, relaxing massage.

Best for: All skin types

0.7 oz	sesame oil	20 g
10	drops coriander essential oil (see tip, below)	10
6	drops sandalwood essential oil	6
6	drops thyme essential oil	6
6	drops orange essential oil	6

1. In a small saucepan, heat sesame oil over low heat just until warm.

2. Add coriander, sandalwood, thyme and orange essential oils. Use immediately for a massage, or let cool, pour into a small glass bottle and seal tightly.

Tip: Another way to enjoy this oil is in the bath. Add a little bit to warm bathwater for an extremely relaxing soak.

Sesame Facial Oil

A few drops of this formula are enough to provide deep moisturizing power. Rub into your face, using gentle circular motions, to help it penetrate the skin.

Best for: Normal or combination skin

1.4 oz	sesame oil	40 g
7	drops cedar essential oil (see tip, below)	7
7	drops sandalwood essential oil	7
7	drops grapefruit essential oil	7

1. Pour sesame oil, and cedar, sandalwood and grapefruit essential oils into a small glass bottle. Seal tightly.

2. Shake to combine.

Tip: Store essential oils in a cool, dark place. Light exposure can diminish their healing properties.

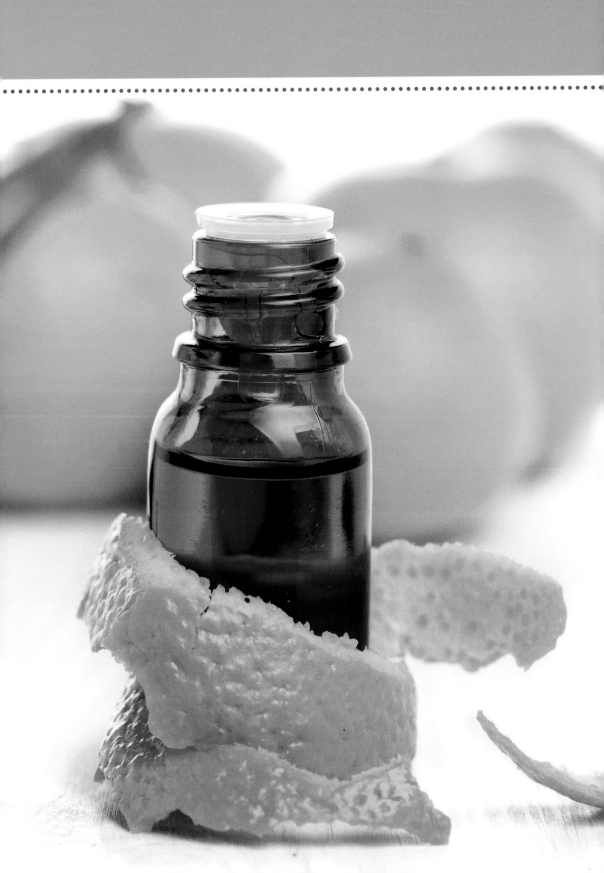

Sesame Energizing Oil

This preparation should be applied during a vigorous massage to activate the healing powers of the oils.

Best for: All skin types

Tip: Instead of using the oil for a massage, add a few drops to a warm bath to boost your energy.

0.7 oz	sesame oil	20 g
10	drops nutmeg essential oil	10
5	drops cardamom essential oil	5
5	drops frankincense essential oil	5
5	drops bay laurel essential oil (see tip, page 79)	5
5	drops patchouli essential oil	5

1. In a small saucepan, heat sesame oil over low heat just until warm.
2. Add nutmeg, cardamom, frankincense, bay laurel and patchouli essential oils. Use immediately for a massage, or let cool, pour into a small glass bottle and seal tightly.

Sesame Anti-Stress Oil

On a busy, stressful day, use this oil to lower your tension level. The best way to apply it is in conjunction with a gentle massage.

Best for: All skin types

Tip: Add a little bit of this mixture to warm bathwater for a stress-reducing soak.

0.7 oz	sesame oil	20 g
20	drops grapefruit essential oil	20
6	drops sandalwood essential oil	6
6	drops vetiver essential oil	6
6	drops petitgrain essential oil (see tip, below)	6

1. In a small saucepan, heat sesame oil over low heat just until warm.
2. Add grapefruit, sandalwood, vetiver and petitgrain essential oils. Use immediately for a massage, or let cool, pour into a small glass bottle and seal tightly.

Tip: Petitgrain essential oil is made from the leaves and twigs of the bitter orange tree. It has a beautiful scent that is different from the scents of orange and neroli essential oils, which are made from other parts of the tree. Petitgrain essential oil is often an ingredient in perfumes.

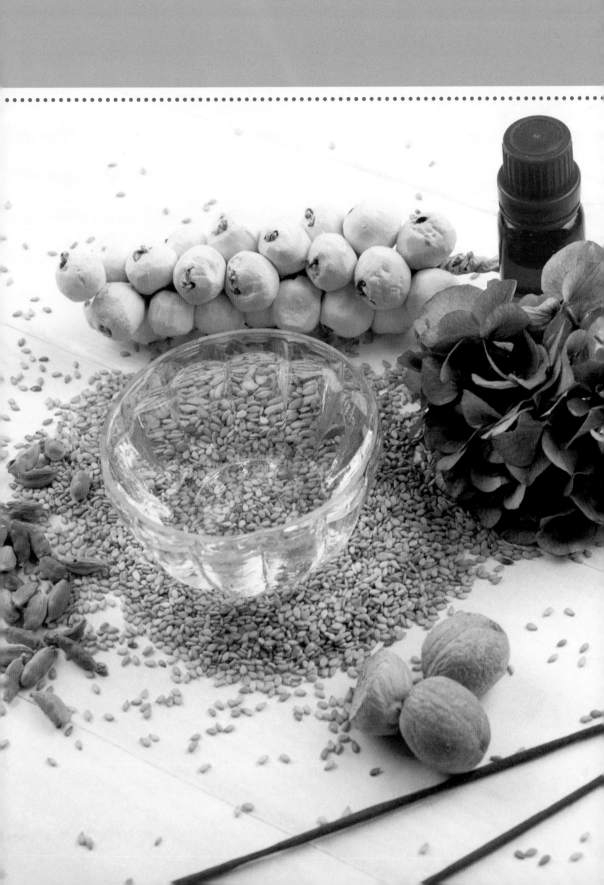

Sesame Anti-Cellulite Oil

Apply this highly fragrant oil once a day to improve the appearance of cellulite. Rub it in with vigorous circular motions until it's completely absorbed.

Best for: Cellulite-prone areas

Tips: The essential oils you use for skin- and hair-care products must be 100% pure. Don't use synthetic scents or oils, or essences used in fragrance burners or lamp rings.

If you have a motorized anti-cellulite massager, you can use this oil with it to intensify its effect.

Note: Exact measurements are important when you're making skin- and hair-care products. Turn to page 17 for how-tos.

5.3 oz	sesame oil	150 g
35	drops lemon essential oil (see tips, at left)	35
35	drops cypress essential oil	35
35	drops rosemary essential oil (see caution, opposite)	35
35	drops fennel essential oil	35
35	drops peppermint essential oil	35
35	drops grapefruit essential oil	35
35	drops cedar essential oil	35

1. Pour sesame oil, and lemon, cypress, rosemary, fennel, peppermint, grapefruit and cedar essential oils into a small glass bottle. Seal tightly.

2. Shake to combine.

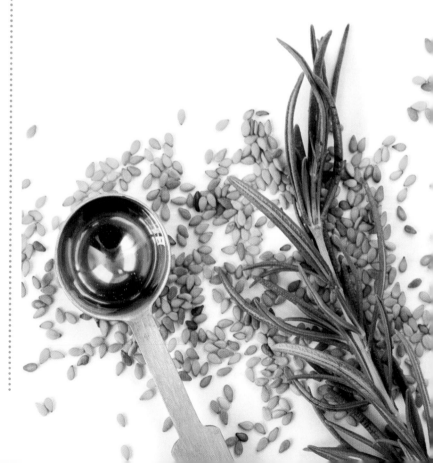

Sesame Flaky Scalp Oil

Soak a cotton ball with this oil and dab generously onto your scalp in areas where the skin is flaking. Cover your hair with a bandana overnight, and wash your hair in the morning. You won't believe the results.

Best for: Dry, flaky scalps

Note: Exact measurements are important when you're making skin- and hair-care products. Turn to page 17 for how-tos.

Caution: Do not use rosemary essential oil if you have epilepsy or high blood pressure.

0.35 oz	sesame oil	10 g
10	drops tea tree essential oil	10
10	drops rosemary essential oil (see caution, at left)	10

1. Pour sesame oil, and tea tree and rosemary essential oils into a small glass bottle. Seal tightly.

2. Shake to combine.

Sesame Oil for a Healthy Smile

There is an ancient Ayurvedic practice of rinsing the mouth with 1 tsp (5 mL) virgin sesame oil. Rinse for a minute or two, then spit it out. Brush the teeth as usual. The oil loosens fat-soluble toxins that are not removed by brushing from the mucous membranes inside the mouth.

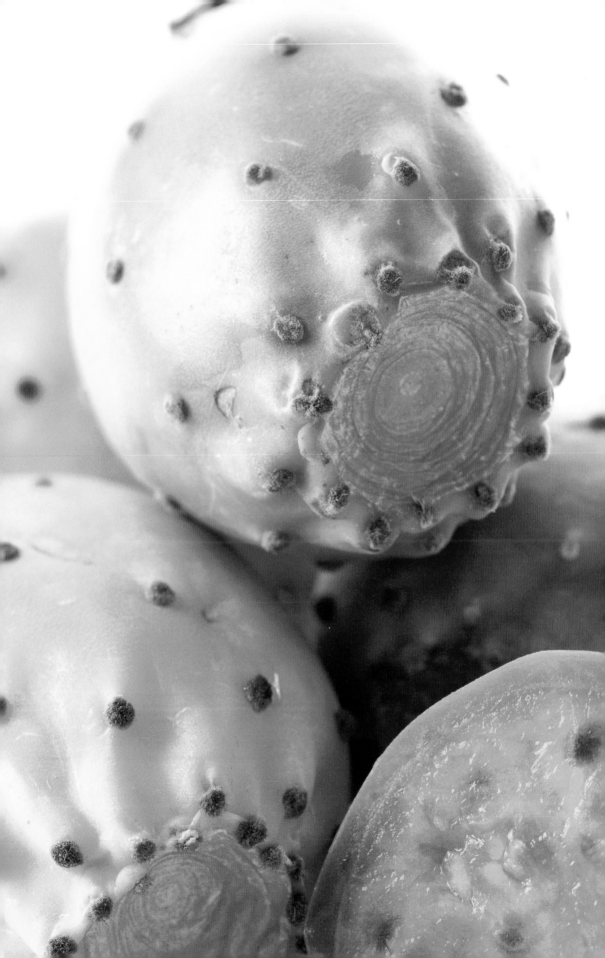

Prickly Pear Seed Oil

This nutritious oil, made from the seeds inside prickly pears, heals and smooths all skin types.

The prickly pear is the fruit of a cactus that belong to the genus *Opuntia*, of the family Cactaceae. The cactuses are plentiful in Mexico, and Spanish conquistadores introduced specimens of them to the Old World in the 1600s. Since then, they have flourished in the Mediterranean region.

Many cultures appreciate the culinary and cosmetic virtues of the prickly pear. From Mexico to Morocco, the fruit is eaten by humans and the cactus flesh is used for animal feed. Prickly pears are rich in potassium, polyunsaturated fatty acids and vitamin C.

Pure prickly pear seed oil is obtained from the seeds that form inside the fruit. (Prickly pear seed oil should not be confused with prickly pear flower oil, which is prepared by macerating prickly pear flowers in vegetable oil.) It takes the seeds of nearly 1,800 lbs (816 kg) of prickly pears to make 4 cups (1 L) of prickly pear seed oil.

This oil has a powerful restructuring action on the skin and is highly nutritious, making it very effective for fighting wrinkles. Its best feature is that it is suitable for all skin types, but at the same time, it is highly recommended for mature and undernourished skin.

Prickly Pear Nourishing Anti-Wrinkle Cream

This rich cream nourishes skin and reduces the appearance of pesky lines on the face. Grapefruit essential oil gives it a fresh, zesty fragrance.

Best for: Dry or damaged skin

Tips: Look for chunks or blocks of pure cocoa butter at cosmetic-supply stores. If you're using a large amount in a recipe, chop it up before adding it to the saucepan so it will melt more quickly.

Look for pure vitamin A in liquid form at cosmetic-supply stores. It's also easy to buy online.

Note: Exact measurements are important when you're making skin- and hair-care products. Turn to page 17 for how-tos.

0.7 oz	prickly pear seed oil	20 g
0.35 oz	hemp seed oil	10 g
0.2 oz	Lanette wax (see box, page 15)	6 g
0.18 oz	cocoa butter (see tips, at left)	5 g
0.15 oz	lanolin	4 g
5.3 oz	mineral water	150 g
2	pinches citric acid powder (see box, page 27)	2
2	pinches ascorbic acid powder	2
0.18 oz	pure vitamin A (see tips, at left)	5 g
20	drops grapefruit essential oil	20

1. Combine prickly pear seed oil, hemp seed oil, Lanette wax, cocoa butter and lanolin in a saucepan. Heat over low heat just until ingredients are completely melted. Remove from heat and keep warm.

2. Pour mineral water into a separate saucepan. Heat until lukewarm. Using a wooden spoon, stir in citric acid and ascorbic acid until dissolved.

3. Stir mineral water mixture into oil mixture. Using a hand mixer, beat at low speed for 1 to 2 minutes. Let stand for 10 minutes.

4. Stir in vitamin A and grapefruit essential oil. Using a hand mixer, beat at high speed for 1 minute.

5. Pour or spoon mixture into glass jars. Let cool.

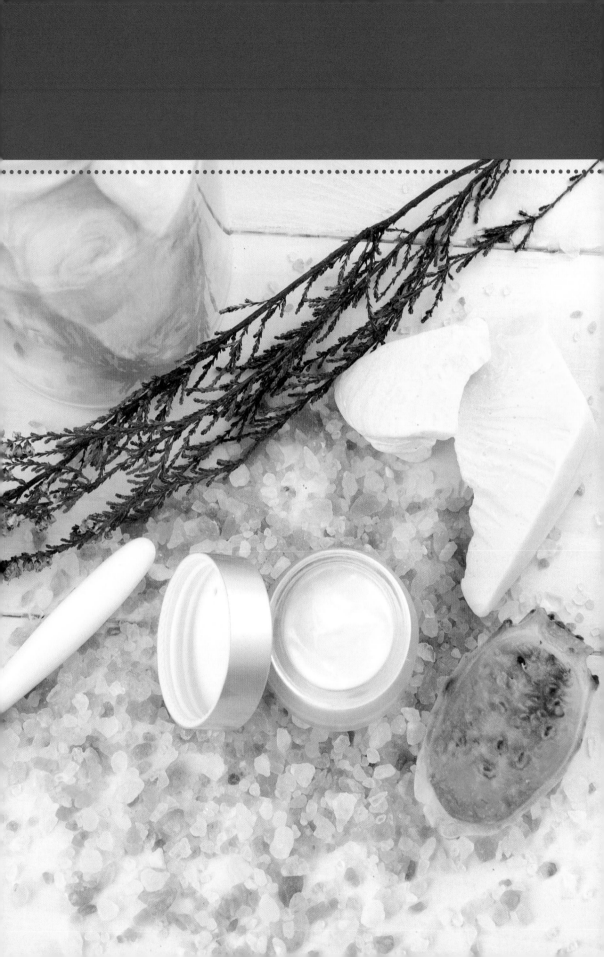

Prickly Pear Anti-Wrinkle Facial Oil

A rich oil like this is an excellent ally in the fight against dry skin and wrinkles.

Best for: All skin types

Tip: Palmarosa essential oil may be a little less familiar than some essential oils, but it has a delicate floral scent that's similar to those of roses and geraniums. It is often used in perfumes.

Note: Exact measurements are important when you're making skin- and hair-care products. Turn to page 17 for how-tos.

0.7 oz	prickly pear seed oil	20 g
0.35 oz	liquid collagen	10 g
0.15 oz	pure vitamin E	4 g
10	drops myrrh essential oil	10
10	drops palmarosa essential oil (see tip, at left)	10

1. Pour prickly pear seed oil, collagen, vitamin E, and myrrh and palmarosa essential oils into a small glass bottle. Seal tightly.

2. Shake to combine.

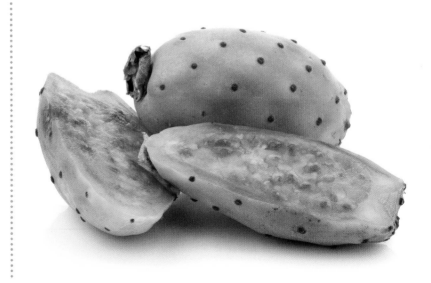

Prickly Pear Extreme Climate Cream

This cream is specially designed for skin exposed to extreme climates, both very cold (such as mountainous and snow-covered areas) and very hot and dry (such as deserts).

Best for: Skin exposed to extreme temperatures

Tip: Lanolin is a waxy natural moisturizer derived from sheep's wool. It has long been used as a softening and moisturizing agent, especially in hand creams. You can find jars of it at cosmetic-supply stores. It has a distinctive, earthy aroma, and a little goes a long way.

Note: Exact measurements are important when you're making skin- and hair-care products. Turn to page 17 for how-tos.

1.8 oz	prickly pear seed oil	50 g
0.35 oz	lanolin (see tip, at left)	10 g
0.2 oz	Lanette wax (see box, page 15)	6 g
4.8 oz	mineral water	135 g
2	pinches citric acid powder (see box, page 27)	2
2	pinches ascorbic acid powder	2
20	drops marjoram essential oil	20

1. Combine prickly pear seed oil, lanolin and Lanette wax in a saucepan. Heat over low heat just until ingredients are completely melted. Remove from heat and keep warm.

2. Pour mineral water into a separate saucepan. Heat until lukewarm. Using a wooden spoon, stir in citric acid and ascorbic acid until dissolved.

3. Stir mineral water mixture into oil mixture. Using a hand mixer, beat at low speed for 1 to 2 minutes. Let stand for 10 minutes.

4. Stir in marjoram essential oil. Using a hand mixer, beat at high speed for 1 minute.

5. Pour or spoon mixture into glass jars. Let cool.

Prickly Pear Neck- and Bust-Enhancing Cream

You take care of your face, but the skin on your neck and chest needs attention, too. Keep it smooth and supple with this silky cream.

Best for: Skin on the neck and bust

Tips: Pure shea butter comes in chunks, like cocoa butter, at cosmetic-supply stores. Break or chop it up before adding it to the saucepan so that it melts quickly and easily.

Hydrolyzed elastin, also called hydrolyzed elastin protein, is a moisturizer often added to cosmetics. It comes in liquid form, and can be found at cosmetic-supply stores.

Note: Exact measurements are important when you're making skin- and hair-care products. Turn to page 17 for how-tos.

1.4 oz	prickly pear seed oil	40 g
0.35 oz	shea butter (see tips, at left)	10 g
0.2 oz	Lanette wax (see box, page 15)	6 g
4.8 oz	witch hazel	135 g
2	pinches citric acid powder (see box, page 27)	2
2	pinches ascorbic acid powder	2
0.35 oz	hydrolyzed elastin (see tips, at left)	10 g
15	drops sandalwood essential oil	15

1. Combine prickly pear seed oil, shea butter and Lanette wax in a saucepan. Heat over low heat just until ingredients are completely melted. Remove from heat and keep warm.

2. Pour witch hazel into a separate saucepan. Heat until lukewarm. Using a wooden spoon, stir in citric acid and ascorbic acid until dissolved.

3. Stir witch hazel mixture into oil mixture. Using a hand mixer, beat at low speed for 1 to 2 minutes. Let stand for 10 minutes.

4. Stir in elastin and sandalwood essential oil. Using a hand mixer, beat at high speed for 1 minute.

5. Pour or spoon mixture into glass jars. Let cool.

Prickly Pear Skin-Repairing Serum

Apply this serum one hour before going to sleep. It will repair and nourish the skin deeply while you sleep.

Best for: Dry or damaged skin

Tips: Snail gel is a relatively new beauty product. It contains a secretion produced by snails that helps them repair and renew their skin. The secretion contains a number of nutrients that are said to be excellent for fighting skin damage in humans, as well. You can find the gel online or at some specialty beauty-product stores.

Look for pure vitamin A in liquid form at cosmetic-supply stores. It's also easy to buy online.

Note: Exact measurements are important when you're making skin- and hair-care products. Turn to page 17 for how-tos.

0.7 oz	prickly pear seed oil	20 g
0.35 oz	snail gel (see tips, at left)	10 g
0.18 oz	rose hip seed oil	5 g
0.18 oz	jojoba oil	5 g
0.1 oz	pure vitamin A (see tips, at left)	3 g

1. Pour prickly pear seed oil, snail gel, rose hip seed oil, jojoba oil and vitamin A into a small glass bottle. Seal tightly.

2. Shake to combine.

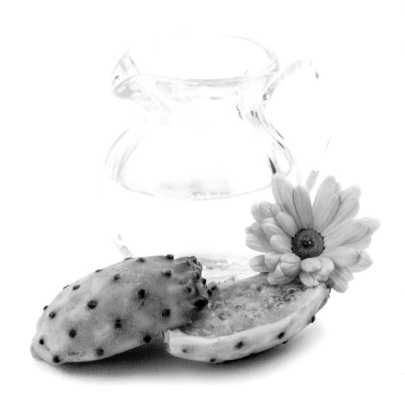

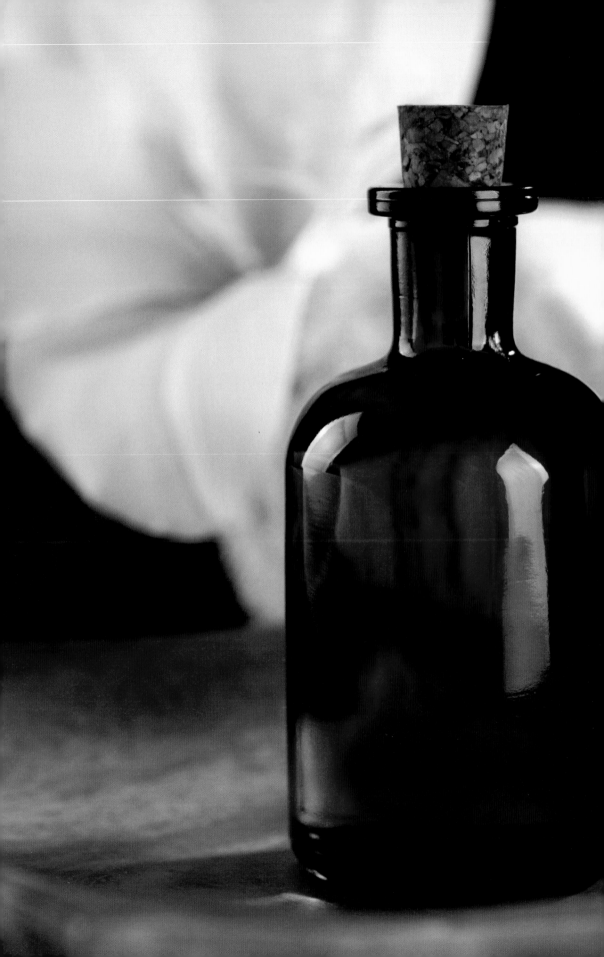

Tamanu Oil

Tamanu oil is used in traditional Tahitian medicine to heal all sorts of skin infections and wounds.

The tamanu tree *(Calophyllum inophyllum)* is native to tropical regions in Asia but grows in many tropical zones around the world. The oil is made from the kernels that form inside the pits of the fruit. The kernels are dried in the sun, then cold pressed to extract the precious oil.

The people of Tahiti have long considered tamanu oil sacred. In ancient times, they created *marae,* or consecrated ceremonial clearings surrounded by stones, where offerings of tamanu oil were made to the gods.

The people of Tahiti have always used tamanu oil in their traditional medicine. It is applied to treat all types of skin infections, even the most serious ones, such as skin ulcers and open sores. Tamanu oil's most notable benefit is its pain-relieving powers, especially for sciatica, lumbago and rheumatism. It is also a natural insect repellent with antiviral, antibacterial and anti-inflammatory properties. It's excellent at fighting wrinkles and free radicals, and is an effective treatment for burns and acne.

Tamanu oil is highly acidic. While it is very effective at treating skin conditions, it should not be used for more than a week at a time, because it can irritate sensitive skin.

Tamanu Insect Repellent

Banish mosquitoes and biting insects without harsh chemicals. Rub a small amount of this oil over arms, legs or any other unprotected areas of skin.

Best for: All skin types

Note: Exact measurements are important when you're making skin- and hair-care products. Turn to page 17 for how-tos.

| 1 oz | tamanu oil | 30 g |
| 10 | drops manuka essential oil (see box, below) | 10 |

1. Pour tamanu oil and manuka essential oil into a small glass bottle. Seal tightly.
2. Shake to combine.

Manuka Essential Oil

The manuka shrub (*Leptospermum scoparium*) is native to New Zealand, where it grows wild, but it is increasingly cultivated in other places. The leaves are hand harvested, and the essential oil is extracted via steam distillation.

In the 1980s, scientists began studying manuka, though its health benefits were already well known to the Maori, who use the plant in traditional medicines. The studies concluded that manuka had many health-enhancing properties, especially for skin. It works in a similar way to kanuka essential oil (see box, page 254), but it is not quite as powerful.

You can use manuka oil as an anti-inflammatory agent to treat sports injuries, or to promote sleep, but you must add it to a base oil. Combine 95% base oil (such as sesame, sunflower or flaxseed) and up to a maximum of 5% manuka essential oil. Mix the two oils together and use the combination when massaging sore muscles or joints. Manuka oil can also be substituted for tea tree essential oil in any skin- or hair-care product recipe, such as foot creams or ointments.

Tamanu Pain-Relieving Massage Oil

This oil relieves pain in the muscles, nerves and joints. Massage over sore areas for considerable improvement.

Best for:
Lumbar, sciatic or rheumatic pain

Note: Exact measurements are important when you're making skin- and hair-care products. Turn to page 17 for how-tos.

Caution: Do not use rosemary essential oil if you have epilepsy or high blood pressure.

1 oz	tamanu oil	30 g
10	drops ginger essential oil (see tip, below)	10
10	drops rosemary essential oil (see caution, at left)	10
10	drops marjoram essential oil	10

1. Pour tamanu oil, and ginger, rosemary and marjoram essential oils into a small glass bottle. Seal tightly.

2. Shake to combine.

Tip: The essential oils you use for skin- and hair-care products must be 100% pure. Don't use synthetic scents or oils, or essences used in fragrance burners or lamp rings.

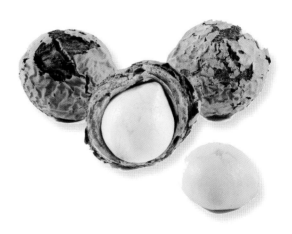

Tamanu Burn-Relief Oil

This oil eases the pain of burns (including sunburns) and scrapes where no infection is present. It is also an effective treatment for chilblains on the feet and even on the ears.

Best for: Burns, sunburns, scrapes and chilblains

0.7 oz	tamanu oil	20 g
0.18 oz	olive oil (see tip, below)	5 g
0.07 oz	lavender essential oil	2 g

1. Pour tamanu oil, olive oil and lavender essential oil into a small glass bottle. Seal tightly.
2. Shake to combine.

Tip: Choose extra-virgin or virgin oils from the first cold pressing.

Tamanu Insect Bite Relief Oil

This oil repels insects and relieves the pain and itching caused by their bites. Using your fingertip, gently rub a little oil onto bites several times a day.

Best for: Itchy, sore insect bites

| 10 | drops tamanu oil | 10 |
| 10 | drops manuka essential oil (see box, page 250) | 10 |

1. Combine tamanu oil and manuka essential oil in a small bowl.
2. Stir to combine. Use immediately.

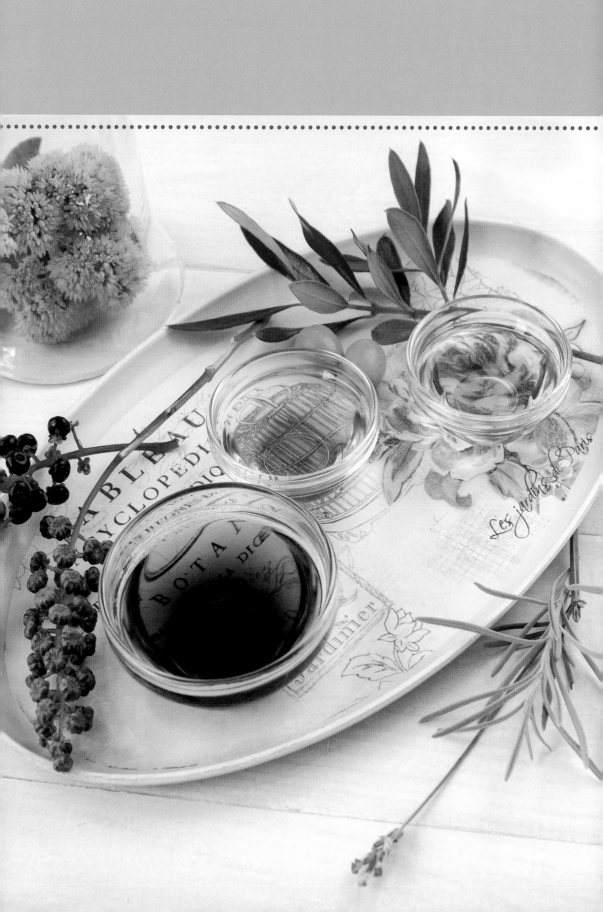

Tamanu
Anti–Cold Sore Oil

Apply this oil only to the affected area. Repeat the treatment three times a day until the cold sore is dry and has reduced in size.

Best for: Active cold sores

Note: Exact measurements are important when you're making skin- and hair-care products. Turn to page 17 for how-tos.

5	drops tamanu oil	5
5	drops kanuka essential oil (see box, below)	5

1. Combine tamanu oil and kanuka essential oil in a small bowl.
2. Stir to combine. Use immediately.

Kanuka Essential Oil

The kanuka shrub (*Kunzea ericoides*) is native to New Zealand. The narrow, pointed leaves are hand picked, and the plant's prized essential oil is extracted from them via steam distillation.

The Maori people of New Zealand have traditionally used kanuka essential oil to treat pain, inflammation and skin diseases. It is more potent than its relative, the famous tea tree essential oil, and even more effective than manuka essential oil (see box, page 250). Kanuka essential oil is antibacterial, antifungal and anti-inflammatory, and promotes deep, restful sleep. It also relieves muscle pain caused by strenuous exercise, repels insects and soothes insect bites.

To kill bacteria or fungi, the oil can be used undiluted. To use it as an anti-inflammatory, to treat injuries or to promote sleep, you must add it to a base oil. Combine 95% base oil (such as sesame, sunflower or flaxseed) and up to a maximum of 5% kanuka essential oil. Mix the two oils together and massage into sore muscles or joints. You can also use kanuka essential oil in place of tea tree essential oil in recipes for foot creams, ointments and so on.

Tamanu Cream for Couperose Skin

This cream is especially recommended for people with couperose skin, a condition characterized by dilation of the capillaries that supply blood to the outermost layer of skin. The dilation tends to cause reddening of the skin, especially on the cheeks.

Best for: Dry and couperose skin

Note: Exact measurements are important when you're making skin- and hair-care products. Turn to page 17 for how-tos.

Caution: Do not use rosemary essential oil if you have epilepsy or high blood pressure.

0.7 oz	tamanu oil	20 g
0.2 oz	Lanette wax (see box, page 15)	6 g
0.18 oz	cocoa butter (see tips, below)	5 g
5.3 oz	witch hazel	150 g
2	pinches citric acid powder (see box, page 27)	2
2	pinches ascorbic acid powder	2
0.7 oz	liquid glycerin (see tips, below)	20 g
10	drops rosemary essential oil (see caution, at left)	10

1. Combine tamanu oil, Lanette wax and cocoa butter in a saucepan. Heat over low heat just until ingredients are completely melted. Remove from heat and keep warm.

2. Pour witch hazel into a separate saucepan. Heat until lukewarm. Using a wooden spoon, stir in citric acid and ascorbic acid until dissolved.

3. Stir witch hazel mixture into oil mixture. Using a hand mixer, beat at low speed for 1 to 2 minutes. Let stand for 10 minutes.

4. Stir in glycerin and rosemary essential oil. Using a hand mixer, beat at high speed for 1 minute.

5. Pour or spoon mixture into glass jars. Let cool.

Tips: Look for chunks or blocks of pure cocoa butter at cosmetic-supply stores. If you're using a large amount in a recipe, chop it up before adding it to the saucepan so it will melt more quickly.

Liquid glycerin is a moisturizing ingredient often included in cosmetics, soaps, shampoos and creams. You'll find small bottles of it at drugstores, but cosmetic-supply stores sell larger bulk amounts.

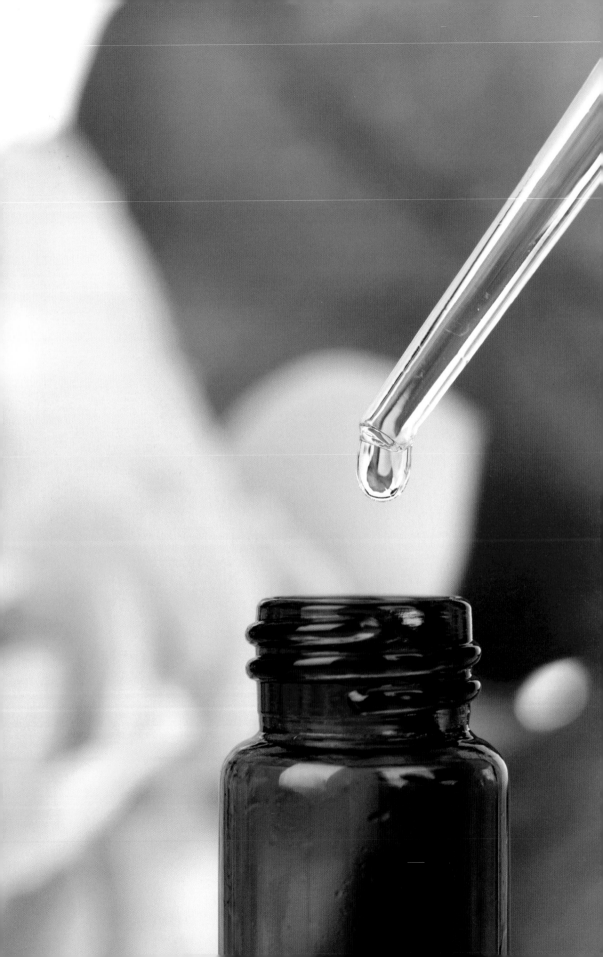

Pequi Oil

Pequi oil is one of the least-known oils used in skin- and hair-care products, but it is a brilliant ingredient in antiaging treatments.

The pequi *(Caryocar brasiliense)* is a shrub native to Brazil. Its oil is extracted from the pulp of the fruit. In the Brazilian countryside, the pulp of the fruit is often eaten, but the oil is used in folk medicine. It is mixed with honey and used to treat bronchitis, the flu and other respiratory ailments.

Pequi oil is rich in carotenes, unsaturated omega-9 fatty acids, vitamin A and lycopene (the same beneficial pigment found in tomatoes). The oil softens dry skin and, above all, helps prevent premature aging of the skin. It is one of the oils that filters and neutralizes free radicals generated by sunlight, so it makes a good addition to sunscreen formulas. It can also help you get a pleasing tan.

Pequi oil is a wonderful healing oil, but it is not well known around the world. It is in short supply, and cutting and selling the shrub are forbidden because the tree is endangered. Production of the oil is therefore carried out completely by hand to ensure sustainability.

Pequi Sunscreen

People with fair skin can use this cream in the winter, when the sun is weaker. People who do not have fair skin can use it year-round for moderate protection. The best idea is to limit sun exposure to avoid skin damage.

Best for: Skin that tans easily

Tip: Look for chunks or blocks of pure cocoa butter at cosmetic-supply stores. If you're using a large amount in a recipe, chop it up before adding it to the saucepan so it will melt more quickly.

Note: Exact measurements are important when you're making skin- and hair-care products. Turn to page 17 for how-tos.

0.35 oz	pequi oil	10 g
0.2 oz	Lanette wax (see box, page 15)	6 g
0.18 oz	walnut oil	5 g
0.18 oz	avocado oil (see tip, page 32)	5 g
0.18 oz	cocoa butter (see tip, at left)	5 g
6.2 oz	mineral water	175 g
2	pinches citric acid powder (see box, page 27)	2
2	pinches ascorbic acid powder	2
0.1 oz	carrot seed essential oil (see tip, below)	3 g

1. Combine pequi oil, Lanette wax, walnut oil, avocado oil and cocoa butter in a saucepan. Heat over low heat just until ingredients are completely melted. Remove from heat and keep warm.

2. Pour mineral water into a separate saucepan. Heat until lukewarm. Using a wooden spoon, stir in citric acid and ascorbic acid until dissolved.

3. Stir mineral water mixture into oil mixture. Using a hand mixer, beat at low speed for 1 to 2 minutes. Let stand for 10 minutes.

4. Stir in carrot seed essential oil. Using a hand mixer, beat at high speed for 1 minute.

5. Pour or spoon mixture into glass jars. Let cool.

Tip: Store essential oils in a cool, dark place. Light exposure can diminish their healing properties.

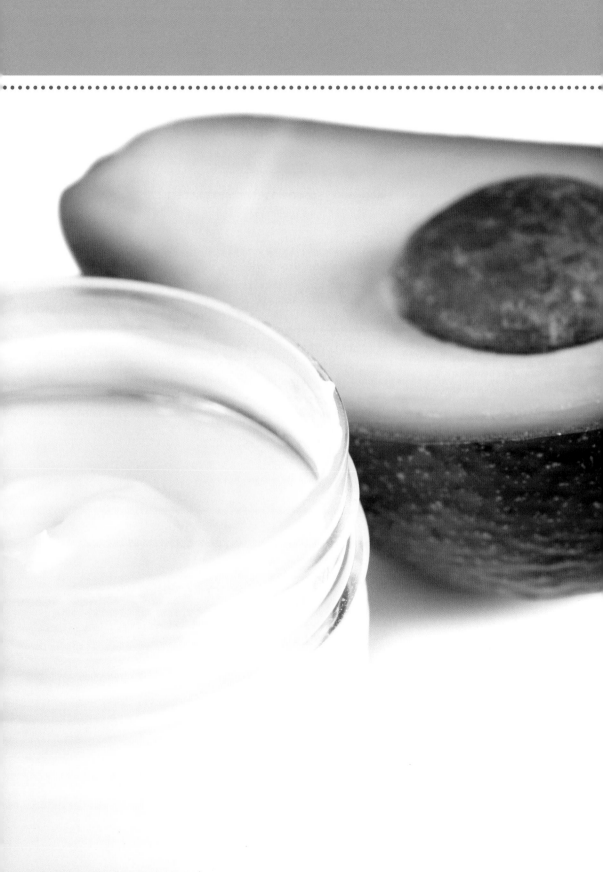

Pequi Firming Body Oil

This oil is excellent for toning and firming skin. Plus, its citrusy, floral, woody fragrance is enticing.

Best for: Loose, sagging skin

Tip: Palmarosa essential oil may be a little less familiar than some essential oils, but it has a delicate floral scent that's similar to those of roses and geraniums. It is often used in perfumes.

Note: Exact measurements are important when you're making skin- and hair-care products. Turn to page 17 for how-tos.

1.8 oz	pequi oil	50 g
1.8 oz	sunflower oil	50 g
0.9 oz	jojoba oil	25 g
10	drops lemon essential oil	10
10	drops palmarosa essential oil (see tip, at left)	10
10	drops cedar essential oil	10

1. Pour pequi oil, sunflower oil, jojoba oil, and lemon, palmarosa and cedar essential oils into a small glass bottle. Seal tightly.

2. Shake to combine.

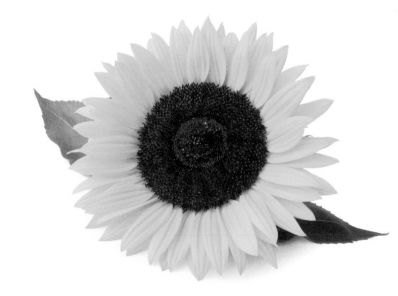

Pequi Anti–Stretch Mark Oil

If you're on a weight-loss plan, this oil can help you avoid developing stretch marks. Massage it into trouble spots daily for best results.

Best for: Areas prone to stretch marks, such as the belly, thighs and buttocks

1.8 oz	pequi oil	50 g
1.8 oz	hazelnut oil	50 g
1.8 oz	sesame oil	50 g
0.07 oz	myrrh essential oil	2 g

1. Pour pequi oil, hazelnut oil, sesame oil and myrrh essential oil into a small glass bottle. Seal tightly.
2. Shake to combine.

Tip: Store the finished oil away from light to keep its healing properties intact. This is a smart policy for all homemade oils.

Pequi and Almond Body Oil

Children's delicate skin needs an especially gentle moisturizer. This oil is perfect for children over six months of age.

Best for: Children's skin

3.5 oz	sweet almond oil	100 g
1 oz	pequi oil	30 g
5	drops petitgrain essential oil (see tip, below)	5

1. Pour sweet almond oil, pequi oil and petitgrain essential oil into a small glass bottle. Seal tightly.
2. Shake to combine.

Tip: Petitgrain essential oil is made from the leaves and twigs of the bitter orange tree. It has a beautiful scent that is different from the scents of orange and neroli essential oils, which are made from other parts of the tree. Petitgrain essential oil is often an ingredient in perfumes.

Pequi and Castor Oil Bath Gel

When you have excessively dry or sensitive skin, you need a soap that won't make the problem worse. This formula cleans the skin but won't remove much-needed moisture.

Best for: Very dry or atopic (hypersensitive or allergy-prone) skin

8.8 oz	rose water	250 g
1.8 oz	glycerin soap base, chopped (see tip, below)	50 g
0.35 oz	pequi oil	10 g
0.35 oz	castor oil	10 g
20	drops geranium essential oil	20

1. Pour rose water into a saucepan. Stir in glycerin soap base. Heat over low heat until soap base is dissolved. Remove from heat and let cool.

2. Stir in pequi oil, castor oil and geranium essential oil. Pour into a bottle or soap dispenser. Shake gently before each use.

Tip: Glycerin soap base is often labeled "melt and pour" in stores that sell soap-making supplies, because crafters use it as the foundation for homemade soaps that are melted and poured into molds. It comes in large bars that range in size from 1 lb to 3½ lbs (500 g to 1.75 kg). Cut off a chunk and chop just the amount you need for the recipe.

Pequi and Cedar Bath Gel

Cedar has a woody, slightly masculine scent, but it's wonderful for women and men alike. Here, it adds aroma to a gentle soap anyone can use.

Best for: All skin types

8.8 oz	mineral water	250 g
1.8 oz	glycerin soap base, chopped (see tip, above)	50 g
0.35 oz	pequi oil	10 g
10	drops cedar essential oil	10

1. Pour mineral water into a saucepan. Stir in glycerin soap base. Heat over low heat until soap base is dissolved. Remove from heat and let cool.

2. Stir in pequi oil and cedar essential oil. Pour into a bottle or soap dispenser. Shake gently before each use.

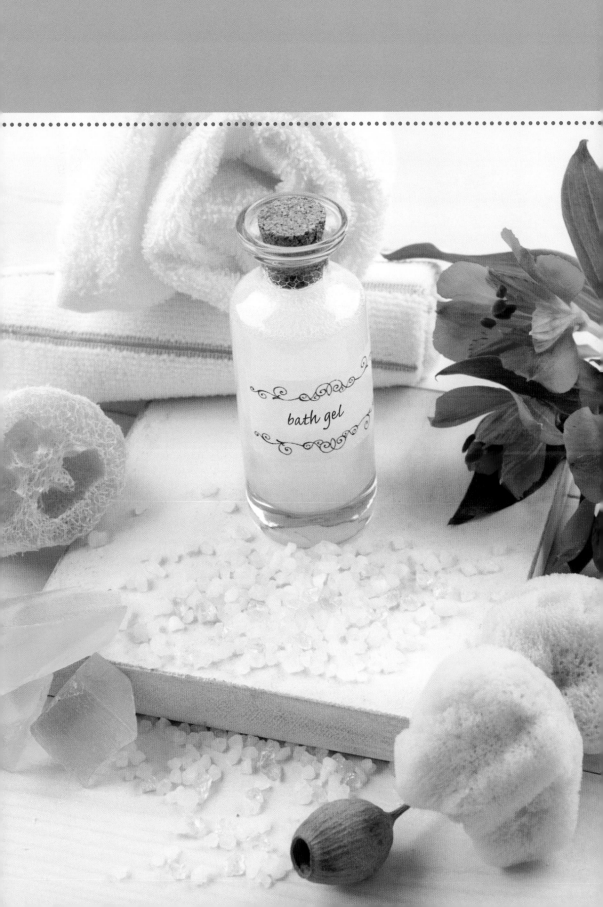

Pequi and Oat Shampoo

This shampoo is especially suitable for hair that is somewhat oily at the roots and drier at the ends.

Best for: Normal or combination hair

Tip: Coco betaine (short for cocamido-propyl betaine) is a surfactant made from coconut oil and gives shampoos their cleaning power and lather. It's easy to find at cosmetic-supply stores.

Note: Exact measurements are important when you're making skin- and hair-care products. Turn to page 17 for how-tos.

2 tbsp	rolled oats	30 mL
5.3 oz	mineral water	150 g
5.3 oz	coco betaine (see tip, at left)	150 g
0.15 oz	pequi oil	4 g
10	drops grapefruit essential oil	10

1. Place oats in a heatproof bowl. In a saucepan, bring mineral water to a boil. Pour boiling mineral water over oats. Cover and let steep for 10 minutes.

2. Using a fine-mesh sieve lined with cheesecloth, strain the oat infusion into a clean bowl. Let cool completely.

3. Pour oat infusion, coco betaine, pequi oil and grapefruit essential oil into a bottle. Seal tightly. Shake gently to combine.

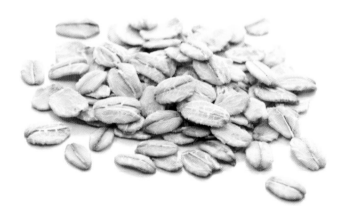

Pequi Nourishing Antiaging Moisturizer

Pequi oil naturally fights wrinkles and dry skin, two telltale signs of aging. The orange flower water base gives the cream a light, fresh scent.

Best for: Skin with signs of premature aging

Tips: Orange flower water is also called orange blossom water. It's easy to find in Middle Eastern grocery stores and some well-stocked supermarkets, where it's sold for use in cooking.

You'll often find two types of chamomile essential oil at cosmetic-supply stores: German and Roman. They come from different strains of the chamomile plant, but both are soothing additions to homemade skin- and hair-care products.

1 oz	pequi oil	30 g
0.2 oz	Lanette wax (see box, page 15)	6 g
0.18 oz	cocoa butter	5 g
5.5 oz	orange flower water (see tips, at left)	155 g
2	pinches citric acid powder (see box, page 27)	2
2	pinches ascorbic acid powder	2
0.15 oz	pure vitamin A	4 g
10	drops sandalwood essential oil	10
5	drops chamomile essential oil (see tips, at left)	5

1. Combine pequi oil, Lanette wax and cocoa butter in a saucepan. Heat over low heat just until ingredients are completely melted. Remove from heat and keep warm.

2. Pour orange flower water into a separate saucepan. Heat until lukewarm. Using a wooden spoon, stir in citric acid and ascorbic acid until dissolved.

3. Stir orange flower water mixture into oil mixture. Using a hand mixer, beat at low speed for 1 to 2 minutes. Let stand for 10 minutes.

4. Stir in vitamin A, and sandalwood and chamomile essential oils. Using a hand mixer, beat at high speed for 1 minute.

5. Pour or spoon mixture into glass jars. Let cool.

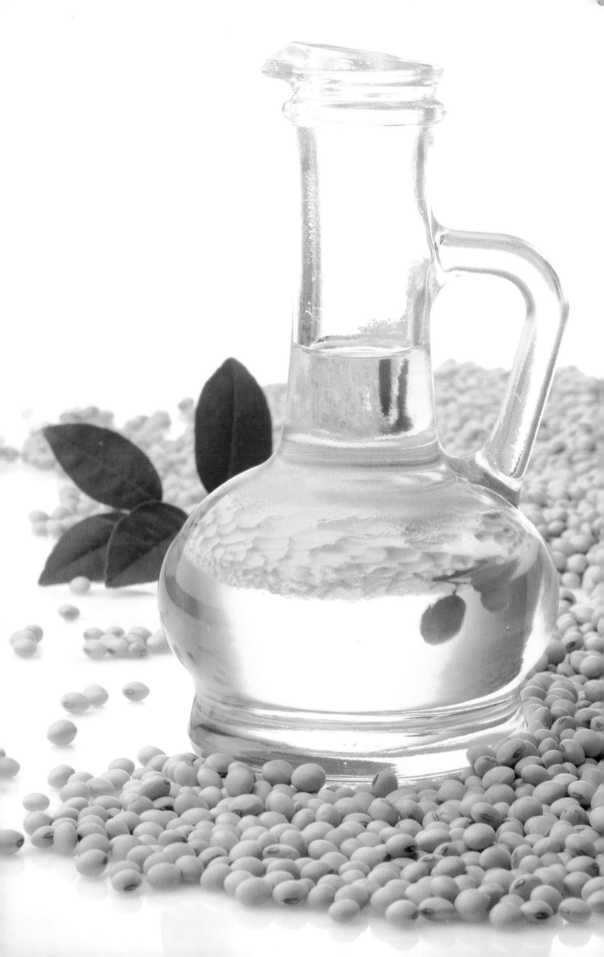

Soybean Oil

The unique feature of creams made from soybean oil is that they leave the skin velvety soft.

There are some 10,000 varieties of soybeans around the world. The most widely used is the yellow soybean *(Glycine max)*, from which soybean oil is obtained. The oil is a common ingredient in Asian cuisine, and is also used in some commercial printers' inks. For cooking and making skin-care formulas, virgin or extra-virgin oil extracted during the first cold pressing is far superior to refined soybean oil.

Soybean oil is rich in monounsaturated fatty acids (omega-9 oleic acid) and polyunsaturated fatty acids (omega-6 linoleic acid and omega-3 alpha-linolenic acid). It also contains phytosterols and vitamin K.

The soybean and food products derived from it — such as soy milk, tofu and soy yogurt — are very popular. Soybean oil is well known in cuisine, but its use in skin-care preparations is not as widespread. Today, there are just a few companies that produce and market cosmetics made with soybean oil — and that's a shame. The oil offers a broad variety of benefits when used topically: it nourishes, moisturizes, regenerates and softens the skin. It is especially helpful in nourishing oily skin.

Citrusy Soy Moisturizing Body Oil

Fight acne all over the body with this refreshing citrus-scented oil.

Best for: Oily or acne-prone skin

Note: Exact measurements are important when you're making skin- and hair-care products. Turn to page 17 for how-tos.

7 oz	soybean oil	200 g
20	drops citronella essential oil (see tip, below)	20
20	drops lemon essential oil	20

1. Pour soybean oil, and citronella and lemon essential oils into a small glass bottle. Seal tightly.
2. Shake to combine.

Tip: Citronella essential oil has a strong lemongrass-like aroma. It's often used in perfumes, and is a natural insect repellent.

Soy Circulation-Stimulating Body Scrub

This exfoliating scrub also stimulates blood circulation. Massage it onto the legs, working from the feet up toward the knees and thighs.

Best for: All skin types

0.9 oz	amaranth (see tip, below)	25 g
0.5 oz	soybean oil	15 g
10	drops marjoram essential oil	10

1. Combine amaranth, soybean oil and marjoram essential oil in a bowl.
2. Using a wooden spoon, stir until ingredients are well combined. Use immediately.

Tip: Amaranth is an ancient grain that's popular in cooking. Look for it in health- and bulk-food stores. The tiny, round grains make an excellent gentle exfoliant.

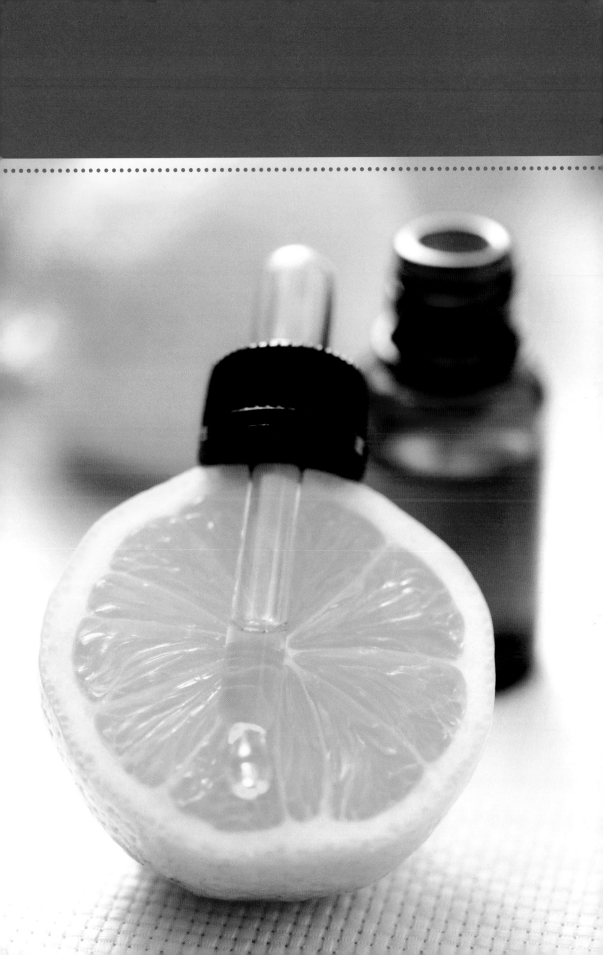

Soy and Hazelnut Slimming Body Oil

Firm, toned skin helps improve the appearance of trouble areas we usually cover up. Apply this slimming oil once a day for beautiful results.

Best for: Areas prone to fat deposits, such as the thighs, hips and arms

Tip: Store essential oils in a cool, dark place. Light exposure can diminish their healing properties.

Note: Exact measurements are important when you're making skin- and hair-care products. Turn to page 17 for how-tos.

3.5 oz	soybean oil	100 g
3.5 oz	hazelnut oil	100 g
35	drops fennel essential oil (see tip, at left)	35
35	drops lemongrass essential oil	35
35	drops sage essential oil	35
35	drops lemon essential oil	35
35	drops cypress essential oil	35
35	drops patchouli essential oil	35
35	drops peppermint essential oil	35

1. Pour soybean oil, hazelnut oil, and fennel, lemongrass, sage, lemon, cypress, patchouli and peppermint essential oils into a small glass bottle. Seal tightly.

2. Shake to combine.

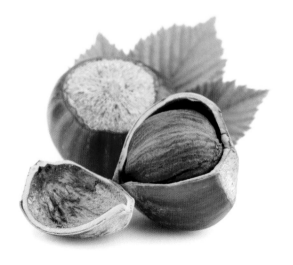

Soy and Rosemary Oil for Tired Legs

Jobs that require hours of standing can lead to exhausted legs at the end of the day. Apply one hour before beginning your workday to stimulate circulation.

Best for: Achy, tired legs

| 3.5 oz | soybean oil | 100 g |
| 0.18 oz | rosemary essential oil (see caution, page 272) | 5 g |

1. Pour soybean oil and rosemary essential oil into a small glass bottle. Seal tightly.

2. Shake to combine.

Tip: You can make this healing oil even more effective by gently massaging it into your feet. This will help boost the relief in your tired legs.

Soy Oil-Fighting Shampoo

Common garden herbs create a fragrant, oil-fighting infusion that's an ideal base for a gentle shampoo.

Best for: Oily hair

Tip: Coco betaine (short for cocamido-propyl betaine) is a surfactant made from coconut oil and gives shampoos their cleaning power and lather. It's easy to find at cosmetic-supply stores.

1 tbsp	fresh or dried sage	15 mL
1 tbsp	fresh or dried rosemary	15 mL
5.3 oz	mineral water	150 g
5.3 oz	coco betaine (see tip, at left)	150 g
0.04 oz	soybean oil	1 g
10	drops lemon essential oil	10
8	drops rosemary essential oil (see caution, page 272)	8

1. Place sage and rosemary in a heatproof bowl. In a saucepan, bring mineral water to a boil. Pour boiling mineral water over herbs. Cover and let steep for 10 minutes.

2. Using a fine-mesh sieve lined with cheesecloth, strain the herb infusion into a clean bowl. Let cool completely.

3. Pour herb infusion, coco betaine, soybean oil, and lemon and rosemary essential oils into a bottle. Seal tightly. Shake gently to combine.

Soy and Rosemary Shampoo

Many people with oily hair and dandruff also suffer from hair loss. This shampoo will treat hair gently, improving its look and feel.

Best for: Oily or thinning hair, and dandruff-prone scalps

Tip: Coco betaine (short for cocamidopropyl betaine) is a surfactant made from coconut oil and gives shampoos their cleaning power and lather. It's easy to find at cosmetic-supply stores.

Note: Exact measurements are important when you're making skin- and hair-care products. Turn to page 17 for how-tos.

Caution: Do not use rosemary essential oil if you have epilepsy or high blood pressure.

3 tbsp	fresh or dried white nettle (see tip, below)	45 mL
5.3 oz	mineral water	150 g
5.3 oz	coco betaine (see tip, at left)	150 g
0.4 oz	cider vinegar	12 g
0.07 oz	soybean oil	2 g
15	drops rosemary essential oil (see caution, at left)	15
10	drops lemon essential oil	10

1. Place white nettle in a heatproof bowl. In a saucepan, bring mineral water to a boil. Pour boiling mineral water over white nettle. Cover and let steep for 10 minutes.

2. Using a fine-mesh sieve lined with cheesecloth, strain the nettle infusion into a clean bowl. Let cool completely.

3. Pour nettle infusion, coco betaine, cider vinegar, soybean oil, and rosemary and lemon essential oils into a bottle. Seal tightly. Shake gently to combine.

Tip: White nettle (*Lamium album*), also called white dead nettle, is a plant native to Europe that has naturalized in many parts of North America. It grows along roadsides and in ditches, which tend to be contaminated by pollution, so it's best to grow your own if possible. Some herbalists' shops carry the dried leaves.

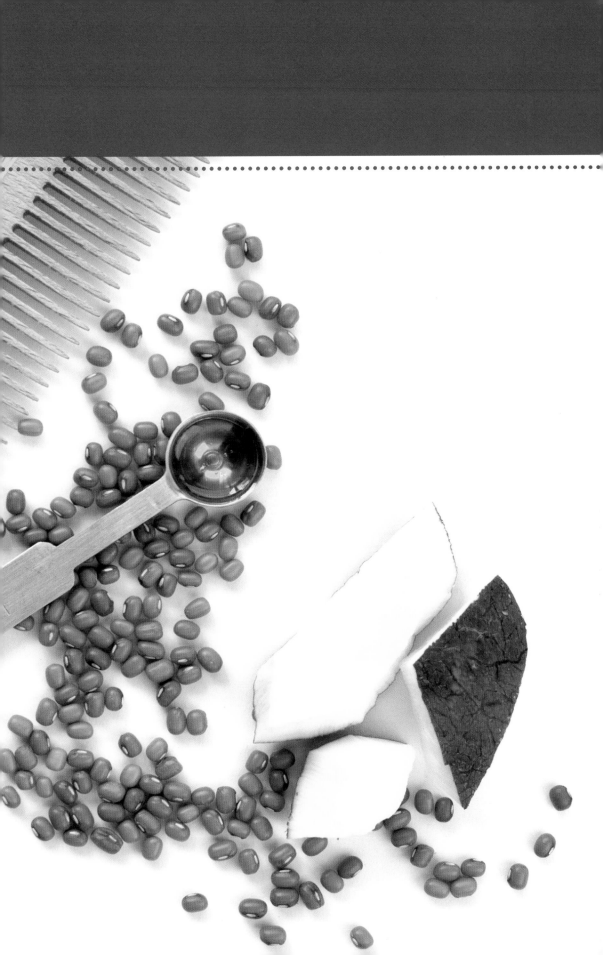

Soy and Jojoba Body Cream

This gentle lotion has everything oily skin needs to keep it vital and refreshed.

Best for: Oily skin

Tips: Rose water is often used in Middle Eastern and Mediterranean cooking. Look for it in Middle Eastern grocery stores and some well-stocked supermarkets.

Liquid glycerin is a moisturizing ingredient often included in cosmetics, soaps, shampoos and creams. You'll find small bottles of it at drugstores, but cosmetic-supply stores sell larger bulk amounts.

Note: Exact measurements are important when you're making skin- and hair-care products. Turn to page 17 for how-tos.

1 oz	soybean oil	30 g
0.4 oz	Lanette wax (see box, page 15)	12 g
0.35 oz	jojoba oil	10 g
12 oz	rose water (see tips, at left)	340 g
2	pinches citric acid powder (see box, page 27)	2
2	pinches ascorbic acid powder	2
0.35 oz	liquid glycerin (see tips, at left)	10 g
20	drops cypress essential oil	20

1. Combine soybean oil, Lanette wax and jojoba oil in a saucepan. Heat over low heat just until ingredients are completely melted. Remove from heat and keep warm.

2. Pour rose water into a separate saucepan. Heat until lukewarm. Using a wooden spoon, stir in citric acid and ascorbic acid until dissolved.

3. Stir rose water mixture into oil mixture. Using a hand mixer, beat at low speed for 1 to 2 minutes. Let stand for 10 minutes.

4. Stir in glycerin and cypress essential oil. Using a hand mixer, beat at high speed for 1 minute.

5. Pour or spoon mixture into glass jars. Let cool.

Soybean Oil Is Terrific for Makeup Removal

Soybean oil doesn't require any additions to make it an effective makeup remover. To remove eye makeup, moisten a cotton pad with water, add a dash of soybean oil and wipe around eyes. To remove makeup on the rest of the face, place a few drops of soybean oil in the palm of your hand and add a bit of water. Rub your palms together to emulsify the mixture, then gently rub over skin to cleanse. Finish by rinsing with lukewarm water.

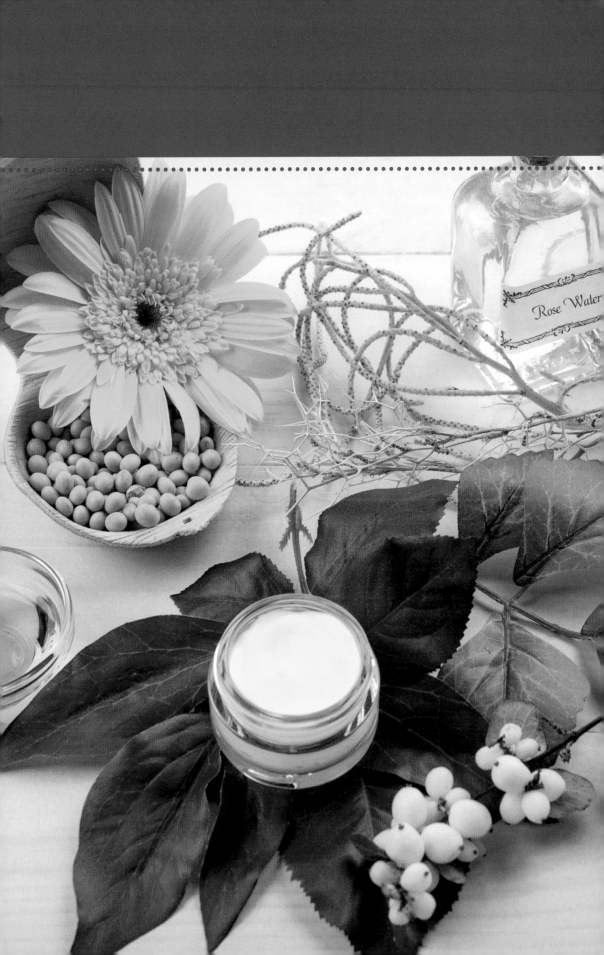

Soy and Kanuka Nourishing Moisturizer

Oily skin may not look like it needs a moisturizer, but it does. This nourishing cream will help skin look and feel balanced.

Best for: Oily skin

Tip: Look for chunks or blocks of pure cocoa butter at cosmetic-supply stores. If you're using a large amount in a recipe, chop it up before adding it to the saucepan so it will melt more quickly.

Note: Exact measurements are important when you're making skin- and hair-care products. Turn to page 17 for how-tos.

0.35 oz	soybean oil	10 g
0.2 oz	Lanette wax (see box, page 15)	6 g
0.1 oz	cocoa butter (see tip, at left)	3 g
6.3 oz	mineral water	180 g
2	pinches citric acid powder (see box, page 27)	2
2	pinches ascorbic acid powder	2
5	drops kanuka essential oil (see box, page 254)	5
5	drops lemon essential oil	5

1. Combine soybean oil, Lanette wax and cocoa butter in a saucepan. Heat over low heat just until ingredients are completely melted. Remove from heat and keep warm.

2. Pour mineral water into a separate saucepan. Heat until lukewarm. Using a wooden spoon, stir in citric acid and ascorbic acid until dissolved.

3. Stir mineral water mixture into oil mixture. Using a hand mixer, beat at low speed for 1 to 2 minutes. Let stand for 10 minutes.

4. Stir in kanuka and lemon essential oils. Using a hand mixer, beat at high speed for 1 minute.

5. Pour or spoon mixture into glass jars. Let cool.

Resources

Associations

Handcrafted Soap & Cosmetic Guild
178 Elm St.
Saratoga Springs, NY 12866, U.S.A.
www.soapguild.org
International nonprofit trade association promoting the benefits of handcrafted soap and cosmetics.

Canadian Guild of Soapmakers, Chandlers & Cosmetic Crafters
www.canadianprofessionalsoap makers.com
Association of professional craftspeople specializing in artisanal soaps and other personal-care products.

The European Directory of Soap and Cosmetic Makers
146 Glasgow Rd.
Longcroft, Stirlingshire
FK4 1QL, U.K.
www.soapmakers.eu
Europe's largest directory of artisans specializing in handmade soaps, candles, cosmetics and personal-care products.

Information

Cosmetic Ingredient Review
1620 L St. N.W.
Suite 1200
Washington, D.C. 20036, U.S.A.
www.cir-safety.org
Supported by the Personal Care Products Council, the U.S. Food and Drug Administration, and the Consumer Federation of America, a panel of experts and policy makers publish safety reviews of ingredients used to make cosmetics.

Supplies

Aussie Soap Supplies
P.O. Box 165
Palmyra, WA 6957, Australia
www.aussiesoapsupplies.com.au
Base and essential oils, cocoa and shea butters, beeswax, soap bases and emulsifying waxes.

Bramble Berry Soap Making Supplies
2138 Humboldt St.
Bellingham, WA 98225, U.S.A.
www.brambleberry.com
Base and essential oils, cocoa and shea butters, beeswax and exfoliants.

Canwax Candle & Soap Making Supplies
114 Lindgren Rd. W.
Huntsville, ON P1H 1Y2, Canada
www.canwax.com
Base and essential oils, cocoa and shea butters, and clays.

From Nature With Love
341 Christian St.
Oxford, CT 06478, U.S.A.
www.fromnaturewithlove.com
Base and essential oils, cocoa and shea butters, beeswax, salts and clays.

Gracefruit Limited
46 Glasgow Rd.
Longcroft, Stirlingshire
FK4 1QL, U.K.
www.gracefruit.com
Base and essential oils, cocoa butter, beeswax, exfoliants, clays, salts, emulsifying waxes and jars.

Healing Spirits Herb Farm
61247 Route 415
Avoca, NY 14809, U.S.A.
www.healingspiritsherbfarm.com
*Bulk herbs, essential oils and
herb extracts.*

Horizon Herbs
P.O. Box 69
William, OR 97544, U.S.A.
www.horizonherbs.com
Bulk herbs, extracts, seeds and plants.

MakingCosmetics
35318 S.E. Center St.
Snoqualmie, WA 98065, U.S.A.
www.makingcosmetics.com
*Base oils, emollients, vitamins, beeswax,
lanolin, emulsifying waxes, citric
and ascorbic acids, and pearl powder.*

Mountain Rose Herbs
P.O. Box 50220
Eugene, OR 97405, U.S.A.
www.mountainroseherbs.com
*Base and essential oils, bulk herbs, cocoa
and shea butters, beeswax, emulsifying
waxes, citric acid and vitamins.*

New Directions Aromatics
6781 Columbus Rd.
Mississauga, ON L5T 2G9, Canada
www.newdirectionsaromatics.ca
*Base and essential oils, cocoa and shea
butters, beeswax, citric and ascorbic acids,
Lanette wax and jars.*

Oregon Trail Soapers Supply
P. O. Box 1456
Rogue River, OR 97537, U.S.A.
www.oregontrailsoaps.com
*Base and essential oils, soap bases,
cocoa and shea butters, beeswax and clays.*

Richters
357 Hwy 47
Goodwood, ON L0C 1A0, Canada
www.richters.com
Bulk herbs, essential oils, seeds and plants.

Saffire Blue
1444 Bell Mill Rd.
Tillsonburg, ON N4G 4G9, Canada
www.saffireblue.ca
*Base and essential oils, cocoa butter,
beeswax and salts.*

Soap Basics
23 Southbrook Rd.
Melksham, Wiltshire SN12 8DS, U.K.
www.soapbasics.com
*Base and essential oils, cocoa and shea
butters, beeswax, clays and salts.*

The Soap Kitchen
Unit 8, Caddsdown Industrial Park
Clovelly Rd.
Bideford, Devon, EX39 3DX, U.K.
www.thesoapkitchen.co.uk
*Base oils, cocoa and shea butters, beeswax,
soap bases and jars.*

Soapmakers Store
Unit 3, Quatro Park
Blakelands Industrial Estate
Tanners Drive
Milton Keynes MK14 5FJ, U.K.
http://soapmakers-store.com
*Cocoa and shea butters, beeswax, citric
acid, emulsifying waxes and jars.*

Voyageur Soap & Candle
#14-19257 Enterprise Way
Surrey, BC V3S 6J8, Canada
www.voyageursoapandcandle.com
*Base and essential oils, cocoa and shea
butters, beeswax, bottles and jars.*

Index

Library and Archives Canada Cataloguing in Publication

Gómez, Mar (María del Mar)
[Cosmética natural con aceites del mundo. English]
    The best natural homemade skin & hair care products : 175 recipes for creams, balms, shampoos & more / Mar Gómez.

Includes index.
Translation of: Cosmética natural con aceites del mundo.
ISBN 978-0-7788-0502-1 (pbk.)

    1. Herbal cosmetics. 2. Hair preparations. 3. Essences and essential oils. 4. Natural products. I. Title. II. Title: Best natural homemade skin and hair care products. III. Title: Cosmética natural con aceites del mundo. English.

TP983.G6613 2015   668'.55   C2014-907383-6